Praise for *Shakti*

"*Shakti Mantras* by Thomas Ashley-Farrand . . . combines his knowledge as an American Hindu priest, [his] adventures as an experienced spiritual guide, [his] considerable storytelling gifts . . . and the immensely practical, useful knowledge of what chants to use when. In his disarmingly unpretentious and accessible style, Ashley-Farrand draws on an enormous body of knowledge from ancient traditions to art and literature and contemporary science. . . . *Shakti Mantras* is an appealingly modest treasure, which everyone—man, woman, young, older, novice, adept—can enjoy. It's as embracing and supportive as a good mother, as entertaining as a teasing sister, and as rewarding as a loving partner."

—DOE LANG, PH.D.
Columnist, DBR Media, Inc.
Author of *The New Secrets of Charisma*

"In the face of difficulty, confusion, or imbalance, there are moments when you may just want to lie in your mother's arms. Thomas Ashley-Farrand's *Shakti Mantras* takes you right to the heart of Divine Mother's energy. From that place of nurturing peace that we all have within, things have a way of working themselves out. What a blessing!"

—IYANLA VANZANT
Author of *In the Meantime*
and *One Day My Soul Just Opened Up*

"Ashley-Farrand throws light on some important secrets. . . . *Shakti Mantras* is a comprehensive work presenting an easily readable account of a range of cultures, mantra practices, and spiritual traditions. [It] provides a wealth of information that can lead to a most rewarding life experience. The mantras are presented in an easy way to pronounce for a Westerner."

—DR. SARASVATI MOHAN
Director, Sanskrit Academy

By Thomas Ashley-Farrand

Healing Mantras: Using Sound Affirmations for
Personal Power, Creativity, and Healing

Shakti Mantras

Tapping into the
Great Goddess Energy Within

THOMAS ASHLEY-FARRAND

Ballantine Books • *New York*

A Ballantine Book
Published by The Random House Publishing Group
Copyright © 2003 by Thomas Ashley-Farrand

Published in the United States by Ballantine Books, an imprint of The Random House Publishing Group, a division of Random House, Inc., New York, and simultaneously in Canada by Random House of Canada Limited, Toronto.

Ballantine and colophon are registered trademarks of Random House, Inc.

www.ballantinebooks.com

Library of Congress Cataloging-in-Publication Data
Ashley-Farrand, Thomas.
Shakti mantras : tapping into the great goddess energy within / Thomas Ashley-Farrand.— 1st ed.
p.   cm.
Includes bibliographical references (p.).
ISBN 0-345-44304-7
1. Mantras. 2. Goddesses, Hindu. 3. Goddesses—Asia. 4. Shakti (Hindu deity)
5. Self-realization—Religious aspects. I. Title.
BL560 .A835 2003
294.5'514—dc21   2002034468

ISBN 0-345-44304-7

Book design by C. Linda Dingler

Cover design by Beck Stvan
Cover photo by GettyImages

Manufactured in the United States of America

First Edition: October 2003

19 18 17 16 15 14 13 12 11

Contents

ACKNOWLEDGMENTS vii

INTRODUCTION 1

1: The Basics—Chakras, Sanskrit, and Shakti 11

2: Saraswati—The Power of Knowledge and Speech 27

3: Parvati—The Power of Consciousness and
    Spiritual Growth 52

4: Lakshmi—The Power of Abundance 79

5: Durga and Chamundi—The Power of Protection 105

6: Kali—The Power of Destruction of Negative Ego 127

7: Lalita—The Great Feminine with a Thousand
    Powers 140

8: Radha—The Power of Divine Love 168

9: Kuan Yin—The Power of Divine Compassion 185

10: Tara—The Power of the Divine Mother 197

11: Misuse of Shakti Power 215

12: Shakti and Your Life 226

APPENDIX: Using Mantras in a Spiritual Practice 235

GLOSSARY 239

BIBLIOGRAPHY 251

Om Sarva Mantra Swarupinyei Namaha
"Salutations to Her who is the source and essential form of all sacred formulas."

—Sri Lalithambika Sahasranama Stotram

"She is the Divine Matrix to whom all of nature dumbly calls."

—Sri Aurobindo

"Kuan Yin . . . is the Mother, the Wife and Daughter of The Logos."

—H. P. Blavatsky, *The Secret Doctrine*

Acknowledgments

I would like to express gratitude to a number of people. I start with thanks to Leslie Meredith, my first editor at Ballantine Wellspring Books, and Tracy Bernstein, my second editor at Ballantine, for their support for my books on mantras. I also want to thank Allison Dickens, my third editor, for her responsiveness and courtesy. Similarly, I thank Stephany Evans of The Imprint Agency for support in many ways, including editing and editorial advice on my manuscript. The Astara organization in Upland, California, has both encouraged my efforts and offered a platform for sharing what I have learned. I am grateful to Dr. Robert Chaney, Rev. Ruby Morrow, and Rev. Steve Doolittle for their support. Joseph Morales has been my webmaster since 1996, when he suggested that I needed a website and offered to put one together for me. I am very grateful.

Others have been very supportive in indirect ways: Rena Elliot-Chiu, a professional psychic and good friend; Suan Yin, a true "sensitive," always ready to help in whatever way is needed; Peggy Rodgriuez, who regularly opens her home for various ceremonies and activities; Nita Johar, who carried my books in her store, Panache, in Claremont, California, when they were no more than photocopied and spiral-bound tomes.

More than anyone, my spiritual teacher and benefactor, Sadguru Sant Keshavadas, deserves credit for this book coming to fruition. He told me in 1975 that I would be writing such books, and

I gave it no credence whatsoever. After his passing, his wife, Guru Mata, has carried on his work, and I am grateful beyond measure for her blessing.

Without the initial suggestion and encouragement by my wife, Margalo, as well as her continuing support, including painstaking editing of a final draft, it is improbable that I would have written this or any other book. Her love is an ongoing inspiration.

Introduction

Mankind has worshiped great feminine archetypes for as long as we have pursued a mystical relationship with life and the universe. The Great Mother, She Who Loves, She Who Instructs, She Who Protects, She Who Heals are but a few of the names bestowed upon the feminine aspect of the androgynous, human nature that we have revered over the centuries. But for most of recorded religious and spiritual history, a decidedly masculine bias has permeated the Western approach to a supreme deity. God is mostly referred to as "He." God the Father is much more often referred to than God the Mother. The great teachers, gurus, and masters have been traditionally represented and described, up until quite recently, as men.

For the most part, until the latter half of the twentieth century, the ancient feminine approaches to divinity were hidden from general public view and teaching. In fact, all the important positions, worldly as well as spiritual, were culturally promulgated to be the province solely of men.

However, with the appearance of the women's movement in the 1960s, a greatly needed adjustment began to take place between masculine and feminine roles in society. In the 1970s and 1980s, a new aspect of the women's movement appeared: interest in woman as goddess. The study of ancient goddess-based religions has flourished since the 1970s and numerous goddess-based books have been written. Since 1990, a flood of books have appeared in both the academic world and the popular press pertaining to something called *tantra*, an Eastern term for tapping into the omnipresent feminine power throughout the universe. Many are listed in the bibliography.

In the late twentieth century, sightings of Mary increased, drawing much more attention to her via television, new books, and worldwide news coverage. And because of this coverage, more people than ever are aware of the sightings and messages of Mother Mary. In the West, we have also become aware of another powerful and active feminine presence in the spiritual realm. Recognition of the Chinese goddess Kuan Yin has spread quickly in the last thirty years and is now revered by more people in the West than live in all of Japan.

Clearly, something is happening to perceptions about women, power, and divinity.

From an objective point of view, a great balancing has been taking place between the sexes as women have begun to understand their own natural power and to move into what have been traditionally male-dominated positions in society. With more women moving into medicine, law, and corporate management, the gender differences in seminars and boardrooms are striking when compared to just thirty years ago.

Things for men are changing as well. A significant number of men have begun to integrate their feminine sides in search of balance. Over the last two decades, many men have begun to feel and understand the emotional needs of children as part of the role of father, and are nurturing their children in an almost maternal way. On television we see men with tears in their eyes or streaming down their faces. Nothing like this would have been possible in the 1950s through the 1970s.

A concurrent trend was seen as we approached the year 2000. From about 1970 forward, the esoteric spiritual and metaphysical movement in this country grew at an extraordinary rate. Almost overnight, literally thousands of people became interested in completely new categories of spiritual subjects. Most of the Western-based, Eastern-oriented spiritual organizations have taken root only since 1970. The Integral Yoga Institute Centers, the Sivananda Yoga Centers, and the Sikh-oriented 3HO organization all have come into existence since 1970. That the changes in consciousness surrounding feminine power and the growth of Eastern-based spirituality occurred together is no accident. The phenomena are intertwined.

Enter the Age of Aquarius

The Age of Aquarius, starting in 2001, can be rightly called the Age of Power. As we moved into the last two hundred years of the Age of Pisces, from 1900 on, we were entering the influence of the new energy that would become the Aquarian Age. As the change in energy approached, we suddenly experienced a dizzying set of breakthroughs relating to power in some way. It is only in the last two hundred years that we have harnessed the power of electricity that ultimately transformed our society from one that used fire-forged tools and horseshoes to the advent of electric-powered factories and computer-driven industries. While the automobile is commonly credited for sweeping changes in our culture, it is electric power that is the real foundation for everything we take for granted in the way we live today. Without it, we would still be stoking up the coals down at the blacksmith's shop instead of plugging in electric-powered forges. We would still be delivering ice to keep food fresh in iceboxes instead of putting food in the refrigerator. With the harness of electricity we soon had the telegraph with its electrical pulses sent down a wire, followed by the telephone, radio, television, and computers. Our lifestyle and business practices start with electrical power. Significantly, the astrological glyph for the Age of Aquarius is the sign of electrical power: two parallel jagged lines that look like lightning.

It is entirely consistent with the astrological view of things that all significant advances in our everyday use of electricity have happened in the last one hundred years, all in the closing moments of the Age of Pisces, as we neared the Age of Aquarius. Astrologers will tell you that we were then close enough to tune in to the energy of the coming age.

The electrical energy indicated by the sign of Aquarius is not just the electricity of the material world, it is also indicative of the powerful feminine spiritual energy that is called *shakti* or *kundalini shakti* in the East. In the West, we often call this energy "spirit." For centuries in the East, water used in religious ceremonies has stood for spirit, the grace and power of the divine to bless us and aid us in coming to grips with life's problems and difficulties.

While the phenomenon of electricity was unfolding in its industrial applications, the influence of shakti, of spiritual electricity, if you will, has also been quietly growing. In the last thirty years, it has burst from its hiding place in Eastern spirituality and come to the West through gurus, lamas, swamis, and spiritual teachers.

The sign of Aquarius is called the Water Bearer. In addition to its symbol of two jagged lines, the sign of Aquarius is often shown as a person—many times a woman—holding a jug of water, indicating that the person is carrying something that flows like water. On the one hand, the astrological Aquarian symbol stands for electricity, while the other commonly accepted symbol shows a person carrying water. Putting the two ideas together, Aquarius can be said to show that a person can carry spirit that flows like water, spiritual electricity. This is not inconsistent with the idea common in the East that the advanced spiritual adept carries and wields the great feminine force called Shakti. Viewed from the

Eastern spiritual perspective, Aquarian energy is spiritual power, shakti power, the power of the Great Feminine.

As we approached the Aquarian Age, it became apparent that the spiritual power of the Great Feminine was not to be confined and hidden. Just as the power of the feminine is moving women forward in society, now it is also pushing out of mystical obscurity and making inroads into the Western spiritual consciousness. Whether discussing the science of electrical energy, or the power of shakti, we are looking at ever-increasing manifestations of power, the power of the Great Feminine.

At the same time, and at least in part because of the increase in the feminine spiritual energy, there has been an ongoing raising of consciousness, described in the East as a masculine attribute. Not only is there a balancing of the two sexes, but we are able to comprehend it consciously and understand it for what it is. To look at it another way, the ideas we contemplate every day are essentially masculine in character because consciousness is masculine. But the "juice," the real power to bring those ideas into manifestation, is feminine.

In the West, we are just catching up to the East in understanding that our masculine consciousness derives its power from the feminine. (More about this in Chapter 2, where the mythic Hindu story of the creation of the universe shows that feminine energy was used to bring a masculine concept into manifestation.)

Why a Man Writes About This

As a Vedic priest, starting in 1973, I have been able, over the years, to watch as these forces have come into play. I have noticed how, from 1970 to 1990, ninety percent of the serious spiritual seekers I met were women. Today it is closer to seventy percent— men are beginning to tune in, to get the idea. As we enter the full effect of the Age of Aquarius, the feminine power has been turned up and its corresponding masculine part, consciousness, has been raised as a result. Women, as natural wielders of power, have been among the first to notice and the first to respond.

Still, you might well wonder why a man is qualified to write about this subject. The answer is that very early in my spiritual practice, my teacher, Sadguru Sant Keshavadas, presented me with the idea that power is a feminine force. He challenged me to prove it for myself. After three years of intense mantra work, much of it centered on the feminine principle, I began to find that there was a force, emanating from the base of my spine, that responded to my thoughts, emotions, and intentions—that force, shakti or kundalini, will be discussed in more detail in Chapter 1.

Nearly thirty years and many thousands of hours of mantra discipline later, I can state beyond any doubt that from my experience, I agree with the seers and sages of ancient India and the teachers who brought the concept of shakti to the West: The nature of power is surely feminine. Through sustained use of feminine-based mantra formulas, the kundalini power of the Great Feminine has introduced herself to me, and as a result I am not the same person I was many years ago. There have been so many positive changes in my life that it is impossible to chronicle them all. The most important change, however, is easy to describe. I came to understand that Love is the greatest power of all, the unifying force for humanity.

Power as Personal Phenomenon

Another important aspect of the Eastern approach is the idea that all power is personal to something. Gravity is personal to the earth, sunlight to the sun, and so forth. But we rarely think of ourselves, human beings, as custodians of power, let alone great power. In the East, however, the concept of personal power is well understood.

The conditions for the acquiring and using of personal power exist in scripture in almost every Far Eastern religion. Demonstrations of personal power by spiritual public figures underline what the texts state. In recent years there have been many reports of spiritual materializations by a swami named Satya Sai Baba, who is said to have manifested many different kinds of objects, as well as a holy ash, called *vibhuti*, before millions of his followers. But it did not begin with him. The modern Eastern classic *Autobiography of a Yogi*, by Paramahansa Yogananda, contains firsthand accounts of many miraculous events. And Yogananda demonstrated his own spiritual power from the grave, as he lay in an open casket for general viewing for twenty-eight days without exhibiting any signs of physical decay.

In classical Eastern texts as well as everyday discussion, personal power of a feminine nature is widely accepted. Paramahansa Yogananda revered "Divine Mother," as he called her. He honored her as the source of all manifested power both personally and in the universe at large. Paramahansa Ramakrishna was totally devoted to his beloved Kali, who was the beginning and end of all power. When Paramahansa Muktananda came to the United States in the early 1970s, he wielded shakti, the awakened and operational feminine power dozing at the base of the spine—yours, mine, and everybody else's. In Muktananda, the shakti was dynamically awake and responding to his conscious direction. People soon began attending his appearances in droves to receive *shaktipat*, the partial awakening of their shakti through the activity of his shakti.

From the time of the appearances of these great spiritual figures in the West, the ancient idea of power as a personal feminine force began to take root here. The practical application of methods to access the kundalini shakti at the base of our spines only began to take shape with the arrival of teachers from India and Tibet who taught various practices, including chanting of Sanskrit mantras or formulas as a foundation for awakening her power.

Following their lead, this book explains routes to manifestations of personal power through the venerable practice of Sanskrit mantra formulas as they relate to the feminine archetypes and their stories.

Keys to Remembering Concepts

It is much easier to read a story and remember the important plot points than to memorize the multiplication tables. Although we cannot remember the finer points from that course in history we liked so much, we can easily sing a song learned in childhood. For the story and the song, a different kind of mental activity sets in that allows us to access the data more easily.

Recognizing this human characteristic, the sages of India constructed stories and fables around great events and concepts. The interaction of the forces of the various planets are reduced to stories where celestial orbs live out melodramatic, soap opera–like stories on a grand scale. The value of this approach to understanding the intermix of great and small forces in the universe is that we remember them better if they relate to a person than if they are a set of attributes of a dry principle.

Further, those sages found that aspects of the Hindu goddesses could be invoked to solve important problems or bless an event. While this is not unlike the goddesses in other cultures throughout history, those with an abiding fascination, attachment, or devotion to any of these goddesses could also invoke the qualities of that goddess into themselves. This is not to say that they would become that goddess. They would retain their individuality. But it was and is possible for you to practice sacred invocations of great power over sustained periods of time so that the qualities and abilities of the goddess are manifested in your life. You can, with work and dedication, take on the very qualities of the goddess herself. This is because the methods to achieve her qualities presume that they all lie within you, material as well as spiritual.

What You Can Get from This Book

There are steps and procedures that enable us to tap our inner resources. We know, for example, that an entire oak tree is contained in an acorn. Down to the last detail of leaf, twig, and trunk, the oak tree exists in a dormant state in the acorn. But through the application of energy acting through time, the tree unfolds from its dormant state. The sublime, alchemical process of photosynthesis blends the energies of sunlight, water, and mineral into a growth process that produces a gigantic tree from the tiny, humble acorn. We know that applying these same energies to a rock will not achieve the same result. It is only because the oak tree is already within the acorn in some form that such a transformation from seed to tree is possible.

Similarly, it is only because the goddess exists in all of us that it is possible to exhibit her attributes and powers. Something cannot come from nothing. The great spiritual attainment by the Indian and Tibetan sages and saints who worshiped the goddess is possible only because she was already within them, as she is within all of us.

To make the attributes, potencies, and methods of invocation for a selection of Eastern goddesses clear and easy to remember, I have adopted the method of classification developed by the Eastern sages—that is, where possible, I tell stories about them. Whether we want to improve our education, bring in abundance, become more attractive, smooth out the wrinkles in our personality, become a magnet for knowledge, a fountain of love, or have some other objective altogether, there is an Eastern feminine archetype representing real, tangible, and usable power that can become available for our use. For each archetype, I tell the mythological genesis and pertinent stories pertaining to her. Then I give mantras you can use to develop within yourself the powers or qualities associated with that archetype.

You can, for instance, become a potent positive force in your work environment with quiet application of mantra power. Your family and work lives can become more harmonious. You can manifest better results in education. You may even get that promotion you wanted. Through the mantra power represented by the great Eastern feminine archetypes, you can learn to manifest desired conditions powerfully and positively. No doubt, you can think of applications, just on the basis of the stories in this book, that would have occurred to no one else.

1

The Basics
Chakras, Sanskrit, and Shakti

If you have a thorough understanding of how mantras work, you may want to skip this chapter. On the other hand, various divisions of shakti are discussed in a way you may not have encountered previously.

Background of Chanting

In my book *Healing Mantras*, I discussed the mystical traditions of many cultures that orally record a rich legacy of tapping into seemingly hidden sources of information and energy through the power of chanting. Some cultures—the Melanesians, Mbuti Pygmies, Cibique Apaches—promote successful hunting and fishing through chanting. Those cultures have used the same methods successfully for hundreds, even thousands of years. But only one tradition has carefully organized and recorded the outcome of chanting in specific ways that is now available to Westerners. To access, bring in, and activate specific qualities of the Great Feminine within, ancient spiritual Sanskrit formulas from India, called *mantras*, can be used with great effect. Ultimately, various types and kinds of the feminine power within, called shakti, can be invoked and activated by Sanskrit Mantra.

The efficacy of chanting specific Sanskrit mystical formulas was carefully hidden and safeguarded by Brahmin priests in India for countless generations. Eventually, however, this information leaked to the secular world, and the use of mantras quickly spun out of control. The power contained in these Sanskrit phrases began to be abused by merchants seeking market supremacy, or by local warlords seeking military success. There was no spiritual foundation for these practices.

Just as the crisis threatened to lurch completely out of control, the Buddha appeared and taught that the Brahmin priests were not needed, the various temples were not needed, and mantras were not needed in order to achieve spiritual and material gain. Within the short span of a hundred years, millions of Hindus converted to Buddhism and gave up the practice of mantra altogether. As a result, thousands of corrupt Brahmin priests found that they could no longer make a living by selling mantra formulas and Sanskrit ceremonies (not unlike the Catholic priests who sold indulgences during the Middle Ages). Many fled to the cities and opened shops, and the great mantra leakage crisis was over.

Of course, even though the Buddha initially taught that mantras were not needed, he eventually did teach mantra practices to various groups. Buddhist sects from Sri Lanka, for instance, have chanted the great Gayatri Mantra for hundreds of years just as the orthodox Hindus do. The great Kalachakra Mantra discipline was the Buddha's final teaching, recorded by only a handful of students who thought they were attending his wake. It is now taught and transmitted principally by Tibetans.

In his book *The Kalachakra Tantra*, the Dalai Lama writes,

"Without depending upon mantra ... Buddhahood cannot be attained."* Clearly, this Buddhist leader places the highest importance on the practice of mantra. If this is the case, what is it about Sanskrit mantras that allows us to tap into some hidden sort of energy? The answer, it turns out, is built into the very spiritual mechanism we inhabit: the chakra system in our bodies.

Our Chakras—Energy Processing Centers

It has been taught for countless generations in the East that another nonphysical, subtle, energy-type body interpenetrates the physical body. The Chinese medical practice of acupuncture is founded on the same idea. In that system, needles are placed in the body at strategic points to aid the flow of energy in the subtle body to diseased or energy-deprived parts of the physical body. In the West, Kirlean photography, developed in the 1970s, captures images of the vibrant light energy emanating from every living thing, whether plant, animal, or human. Kirlean photographs have been taken of the energy emanating from the hands of healers. In its higher and more developed phases, this energy is responsible for the nimbus or halo surrounding certain saints and sages throughout religious history.

It is the energy coming from the subtle body that provides the key to the effectiveness of Sanskrit mantra chanting.

Similar in structure to the physical body, the subtle body has a spine through which energy flows and, through tubes similar to veins and arteries, called *nadis* in Sanskrit, is eventually distributed to all parts of the subtle body. Located along the spine in the subtle body are whirling energy processing centers called *chakras*

*Dalai Lama XIV [Tenzin Gyaltso] and Jeffery Hopkins, *The Kalachakra Tantra* (Boston: Wisdom Publications, 1992), page 165.

that correspond in location to the major nerve ganglia (cervical plexus, solar plexus, sacral plexus, and so forth) located along the spine in the physical body. To those who can see their workings, the chakras look like spinning pinwheels, which accounts for their name in Sanskrit, meaning wheel. To others, the chakras look like flowers, each possessing a different number of petals.

In healthy people, the chakras are vibrant and spin with vigor, facing out from the subtle spine. In those who are not well or who have abused themselves through drugs or alcohol, the chakra flowers are dull and spin sluggishly as they hang facing downward, listless and only partially active.

The ancient Indian mystics with "second sight," the ability to see clearly into the subtle realm, noticed that when certain Sanskrit syllables were pronounced, certain petals on some chakras responded very positively. For an indeterminate time, mystical mantra experiments were conducted and their results passed on orally to successive generations of spiritual teachers. Results of early experiments were verified as practitioners used mantra formulas identical to some of the early seers and found, amazingly, that later users of those same mantras all arrived at a nearly identical state of being.

Those ancient seers also noticed that when certain Sanskrit sounds, not all of which were words or meaning-based sounds as in modern language, were chanted in certain sequences, the resulting vibrational effect upon the chakras and physical body was remarkable. The sounds seemed to work synergistically, producing significant results in whoever chanted them, whether they understood what they were chanting or not.

The more the mystics investigated through expanded means of subtle perception, the more they understood what was happening. They saw that we are surrounded by energy all the time: spiritual energy. They also saw that when the Sanskrit formulas were chanted—that is, as the petals on the chakras vibrated in mystical resonances—a tiny amount of this spiritual energy was actually pulled into the subtle body. The chakras were accessing and drawing in the energy that surrounds us all the time. One may say by way of analogy that our chakras were little TV sets that, instead of pulling in television signals, pulled in spiritual energy. Continuing this analogy, the various chakras are the different channels. By the chanting of the Sanskrit formulas, people were experiencing a net gain not just in energy but in *usable* spiritual energy.

Over months and years of such activity, the energy gains were amazing. People who previously had no noticeable aura now had one. Among those who had been seemingly quite ordinary, some became healers, while others seemed to grow wise and mysteriously tap into realms of spiritual knowledge and understanding. The total amount of energy in the body was increasing as chanting continued over time, because the chakras were constantly accessing, pulling in, and processing new energy.

So astonished were these early seers that they acted just like the CIA of today. They immediately clamped a lid on the spread of this knowledge even as they continued to study it. As the years rolled by, the sages noticed that continuous chanting led to spiritual abilities, such as clairvoyance (mystical seeing), clairaudience (mystical hearing), as well as others. The subtle body, as it grew, began to work with the laws of the universe in ways that seem like science fiction today. These outcomes were carefully written down (after the advent of writing) and can be found today in the *Vedas*, the *Upanishads*, and most recently the *Yoga Sutras of Patanjali*.

Finally, the sages arrived at an understanding of how the energy-gaining process of the chakras was directly tied to the Sanskrit language. The six chakras located along the spine of the subtle body each have a different number of petals—or spokes, if you prefer. The total number of petals or spokes composing those six chakras is fifty. Similarly, the Sanskrit alphabet consists of fifty letters, with each one corresponding to a particular petal of a chakra. When a mantra built from the language is chanted, our chakras vibrate in tune with the Sanskrit sounds because Sanskrit is specifically vibrationally tuned to the activity of our chakras. Sanskrit is an energy-based language first and a meaning-based language second. It is not only the language of our chakras, it is a language that the feminine-based power within us understands, and to which it also responds.

Shakti Power

In numerous texts on yoga, meditation, and Eastern mysticism, we find references to different types of shakti power—the Great Feminine energy that exists both within and without our bodies.

As a force in the universe, shakti powers everything, from the planets in their orbit to the radiant power of the sun. Whether referring to the power behind gravity or the power behind the speed of light, shakti is the term used to describe the operating power of the cosmos, from the smallest atom to the grandest galaxy. Any kind of force, power, or influence has its genesis in shakti, and shakti is feminine in nature.

In us, shakti is described in innumerable mystical texts as a serpentlike power cell coiled three times, sitting at the base of the spine. This atomic-like power cell furnishes the energy we use for both conscious and subconscious functioning. The housecleaning our bodies perform while we sleep is powered by the shakti that energizes the sympathetic, parasympathetic, and autonomous nervous systems to send instructions to the lymphatic system, the pituitary gland, and a host of other places in our slumbering forms. Whether it is blood circulating in the veins and arteries, a nerve impulse jumping a synaptic gap in the brain, our body straining while running the hundred-meter dash, or the working out of a physics or organic chemistry problem, our shakti provides the energy to accomplish the activity. Since many of these functions go on all the time behind our consciousness, we don't think about them. But aware of it or not, shakti is the power behind them all.

Throughout many lives, the higher spiritual purposes of this great power begins to manifest. The shakti sitting at the spine's base will eventually unfold itself and send its essence, energy, up the spine to the top of the head. Along the way, it activates the chakras in certain mystical ways, and pierces successive veils of ignorance, in the form of knots (called *granthis* in Sanskrit) that are strategically placed along the spine to protect us from premature access to higher realms and spiritual states. No matter who we are or what our station in life, the adepts who see such things report that the knots are in the same place in every person.

Finally, over the flow of successive lives, as the energy reaches the top of the head, we will have exhausted every kind of karma in every realm and become completely liberated.

Classifications of Shakti Power

Different spiritual texts describe different kinds or classifications of Shakti power, such as references to Jnana Shakti or Iccha Shakti. Or we may read about Kriya Shakti or Para Shakti. But it is only in H. P. Blavatsky's *The Secret Doctrine*, written early in the twentieth century, that we find all categories and divisions of shakti clearly defined. I've paraphrased these definitions below.

Para Shakti

Para Shakti is the Supreme Force that exists throughout the entire manifest universe. Scientists have been carefully studying its principal attributes, heat and light, for as long as we have inquired about the nature of the cosmos. But for all its investigation, modern science knows only a little about light. It cannot even be said with certainty if it is a particle or a wave. But we can measure many of its physical properties. The same is true of heat. Whether measuring heat on the Earth, on the moons of other planets, or way out in the galaxy, we generally know how hot or cold things are. However, with regard to "spiritual" light and heat, we have very little in the way of scientific data, because there are no mechanical tools available to study or measure these phenomena. Spiritually speaking, the light of the aura is a manifestation of Para Shakti. Similarly, the Tibetan practice of generating intense body heat, called *tummo*, is Para Shakti in action.

Jnana Shakti

Jnana Shakti is the power of the intellect, of real wisdom, of which there are two main divisions. The first involves essential attributes of the mind. The self-aware mind can recall previous events and activities through the faculty of memory. It adds to the richness of understanding through the use of data that comes from the senses. To do this, the mind categorizes things into coherent groups that are analyzed and then stored either in short-term or long-term memory. Recognizing itself as a separate entity in the universe, the mind considers differences between itself and external objects and conditions. All of these fall into the category of the feminine power that activates the mind to perform these tasks: Jnana Shakti

The mystics also speak of the nonmaterial attributes of the mind that are powered by Jnana Shakti, such as the ability to understand events that seem to transcend time and space. When Edgar Cayce was able to send an ill person to an obscure location to procure a medicine hidden on a shelf behind bottles in front of it, Jnana Shakti powered this nonmaterial ability. Any real ability of clairvoyance or clairaudience is powered by this shakti.

Iccha Shakti

The power of will, Iccha Shakti is something we often associate with making decisions and then sticking to them. But there is really much more to it than that. When we decide to pick up an object, a series of events takes place. The mind sends thought instructions via nerve paths to a group of muscles that receive the commands and then begin to operate in the way they were told. All of these activities use energy. First, there is the energy of original thought, then comes the energy of the thought transmission to the nerves that subsequently travels on to the muscles themselves; finally, there is the action of the muscles themselves. Iccha Shakti fuels all of these.

Through Iccha Shakti we move from place to place through locomotion. We manipulate objects with our hands. With Iccha Shakti, we harness the power of Jnana Shakti, the mental power, by means of the muscles in the throat and voice box to communicate and influence one another through speech and song. Healers send life energy, *prana* in Sanskrit, to their clients through Iccha Shakti when they lay hands on or over a client. Iccha Shakti, as willpower, is a type of power separate from the purely cognitive powers covered by Jnana Shakti.

Kriya Shakti

This is the mysterious power of manifestation. Through this power, acting in combination with Jnana Shakti, we create art and music and can achieve creative synthesis for new advances in any field. Although there is a fine line between intuition, a function of Jnana Shakti, and creativity, a function of Kriya Shakti, it is the latter that is the source of manifestation. In the current era, the power of manifestation demonstrated by Sai Baba in India and other lesser-known spiritual figures is directly tied to this type of shakti. We can use this shakti in conjunction with other types of shakti to create new conditions in our life such as wealth and good health.

Kundalini Shakti

Kundalini Shakti is the power inherent in nature. It includes the phenomenon of electricity and magnetism. Esoterically, it is the shakti that matches our internal conditions with an external reality, which means that it is a pivotal factor in determining the conditions and circumstances of our rebirth according to something called our karma, discussed later in this chapter. Since our internal karmic condition is always matched to circumstances of our birth, including country and community and the kind of family into which we are born, this shakti is always in tune with the changing nature of our karma, day to day and life to life.

Mantra Power

Mantra Shakti is unique in that it can be used to invoke and build within you the abilities and characteristics of the other five types of shakti. Specific Sanskrit mantras can produce states and effects that are unmistakable manifestations of the other types of shakti.

For instance, by saying a certain kind of mantra, one can set forces into motion that will increase memory power. For centuries, people in India have chanted Saraswati (Chapter 2) mantras to achieve better results in school. This is an activity of Jnana Shakti that has been activated by mantra. Or one might desire a better home and chant mantras invoking the power of Lakshmi (Chapter 4), activating Kriya Shakti.

The fact that Mantra Shakti can be used to invoke and develop all the other kinds of shakti underscores the importance of Sanskrit mantras in solving most of the problems we confront in life. Our karma may be embedded, like the root of a wart that goes deep into the flesh, taking great effort to move it aside or balance its momentum. Still, it can be done, and great changes can be wrought in our lives in the midst of seemingly impossible conditions. Large-scale changes can be achieved through dedicated mantra effort combined with consistent practice. If we are determined and disciplined, we can solve huge karmic problems and overcome persistent undesirable conditions.

Inner and Outer Shakti

To accomplish our spiritual and material objectives, we need to understand the relationship between the inner shakti, sitting at the base of the spine, and the outer abundance of energy that exists in states represented by the first five divisions of shakti.

In spiritual development, new rules governing the relationship between internal and external power begin to appear as a seeker advances. In fact, something amazing happens when certain levels of spiritual development are reached. As the practitioner works with mantra over days, months, and even years, the steady accumulation of energy that was discussed earlier takes place. The subtle life energy, prana, grows more vibrant and powerful. All the chakras work to provide more energy in finer and finer gradations to all parts of the spiritual/physical mechanism.

At some point, the intelligent shakti power cell at the base of the spine becomes aware that the energy-carrying potential of the spiritual body has increased. If our capacity was, say, a ten-watt bulb, now it has become a twenty-five-watt bulb. All the spiritual work with mantra has steadily increased the available and usable spiritual energy in the subtle body. At the same time, the ability of the subtle body to use even higher amounts of "voltage" has also been increased by the mantra work. Accordingly, the shakti releases increased amounts of energy into the spine in the subtle body. Because our capacity has increased, shakti gives us more energy with which to work: a *second net gain* in usable spiritual energy.

In essence, our work to produce one kind of gain has produced an effect that also generates another kind of net gain. This means that all the mantra practices you perform will have not just one result but *two* over the course of time. By this route, an initial ten-watt bulb can eventually grow to carry fifty, one hundred, or even five hundred watts of spiritual charge. These highly charged human bulbs among us are the great spiritual teachers around whom organizations and movements form. Those with even greater charges have entire religions formed around them. But all of these leaders say that what they have attained, we can also attain. This is a truly powerful potential outcome from your dedicated mantra discipline.

Other Methods

In the spirit of inclusion, Sanskrit mantra is not the only way to awaken our kundalini.

Sincere prayer will, after some time, depending upon the depth of the supplicant's sincerity, begin to arouse one or more of the various types of shakti.

Hatha Yoga, practiced under the leadership of a qualified teacher, will produce conditions in the body where kundalini activity will occur.

Music is very powerful in producing ecstatic states resulting from kundalini activity, particularly if that music comes from a master musician, such as Ravi Shankar, or a master composer, such as Mozart.

The various yogas—Jnana, Bhakti, Raja, Karma, Kriya, Laya, as well as Hatha—can all produce states conducive to shakti activity.

A very advanced spiritual teacher can awaken our kundalini through mystic means at his or her disposal, but this is not an everyday occurrence, even if we should be so fortunate as to meet such an advanced teacher.

Very occasionally, our past good karma will manifest as a shakti experience of one type or another. But even in these cases, people are hard-pressed to find a way to cause the experience to reoccur.

Sanskrit mantra is an easy way to systematically awaken and harness the Great Feminine shakti that sits waiting to be invoked and invited into the center of our lives. Paramahansa Yogananda would tell people, "Call to Divine Mother, because the Mother is nearer than the Father." Through Sanskrit mantra, we are calling to the Mother in a language she easily understands.

Karma

There is one more topic to touch upon before we discuss specific kinds of shakti and how to invoke them into your life: karma.

Most of us question the reasons for some of the circumstances in our lives that appear, often suddenly, seemingly out of nowhere.

Why did I get sick at just the wrong time?

Why did that job I wanted go to someone else when I was better qualified?

Why did they say those things about me? I never did anything to them.

We have all asked these and similar questions from time to time. In the Western psychological model and scientific way of thinking, there is no way to explain the causality of such events other than by random chance. In Eastern philosophy, however, the cause of all these kinds of things is placed in our karma.

The idea of reincarnation, the soul living more than once, is central to understanding the functioning of karma. Using a concept identical to "as you sow, so shall you reap," the Law of Karma holds that consequences of actions in one life can return in subsequent lives. Since we have lived many times, we may have lots of consequences of past actions, or karma, to balance or work out. Because for most of us the amount of karma we have is quite large, only a certain, specific amount of karma is destined to be worked out in any one of our lifetimes. In its simplest form, karma is the Law of Cause and Effect of all our thoughts and actions stretched over more than one lifetime.

If something undesired occurs in your life, the Law of Karma would posit that you did something in a previous life that produced the undesired result in this lifetime. What you sowed in a past life you are now reaping in the present one. Good karma works the same way. When something unexpectedly good happens, you are said to have "good karma." Your good actions in a previous life made deposits of good fortune in your karmic bank account and now you are reaping dividends.

The idea of karma gives new meaning to life instructions embedded in the Ten Commandments, or Jesus' dictum to "love one another." Following these prescriptions for behavior produces good karma automatically. The phrase "what goes around comes around" also expresses the idea of karma. The Eightfold Path of the Buddhists, which includes such items as "right thinking" and "right livelihood," is similarly intended to create good karma.

Ultimately, the goal is to balance or work out all our karma. When we have achieved this, we are "free," spiritually speaking, of any indebtedness on the Earth plane and can move on to other realms of existence.

From Whither Come the Realms?

The Vedas are the world's oldest scriptures. They are written in Sanskrit and predate any of the modern religions. According to the Vedas, there are many realms scattered through many dimensions. String theory in modern physics echoes these ancient ideas, posing the possibility of numerous dimensions of reality. But where do they all come from initially? And more pertinently, what is the genesis of this universe?

Contemporary physics generally accepts the "monoblock" theory of creation. Simply put, this theory holds that originally all of the matter in our known universe was compacted into a single mass at one location. The force of such a great mass concentrated in one place produced an explosion the magnitude of which is beyond our ability to comprehend: the Big Bang. Flinging matter in all directions at a velocity close to the speed of light, the universe as we know it was created.

As matter began to cool and coalesce, suns and planets and galaxies were formed, and life came into being. Given the laws of physics as we currently understand them, there will come a time far in the future when the original impetus generated by the explosion of the monoblock will be exhausted. Matter will have slowed its headlong flight into the night of nothingness and eventually halt. During this running down and dispersal of all the matter and energy in the universe, which science calls entropy, suns will expand in a dying gasp and consume their planets and then wink out one by one, even while black holes increase their size and engulf stars and whole galaxies. Essentially, the universe will come to an end.

You may have noticed that something is missing from this theory. Where did the monoblock come from? Science as we know it holds that something cannot come from nothing, so where does this colossal hunk of matter come from? The answer is, we don't know.

But if science has not yet been able to answer the really big questions, we do at least have the venerable spiritual texts and teachings from the Vedas and Puranas of ancient India. The Puranas are sweeping myths, stories, and fables that explain the very origins of matter and the genesis of the universe through characters in a huge drama. Through these stories, the creation of the soul, or *atman*, is also portrayed.

The next chapter will contain the story of the creation of the universe though the interaction of Narayana, Lakshmi, and Brahma, long before the dawn of time.

2

Saraswati
The Power of Knowledge and Speech

In the East, the power of knowledge, the active force behind any mental process, is the feminine archetype Saraswati, an energy that empowers the mind through the chakra at the brow center. She also presides over speech. Activated by shakti but residing in us as a force emanating from the chakra at the throat, the pinnacle of her power through speech is Sanskrit mantra.

Invoking her power into our mind, we can solve great mysteries or take ideas and activate them through the power of speech. Saraswati also empowers anything relating to music. Whether musician or composer for secular music or spiritual hymns, Saraswati is the force of inspiration as well as performance.

Long the hidden force behind Eastern spirituality, Saraswati is widely revered by Hindu swamis as well as Tibetan lamas. The powers she bestows through disciplines pertaining to her are impartial. Any person can invoke her power into events and circumstances. Chanting mantras that activate her power can result in becoming a vehicle for her Grace.

In the West, we are familiar with affirmations, where we read and speak a powerful idea that positively programs our subconscious mind. This is the power of Saraswati with which we are more familiar. Catherine Ponder's books on self-healing and generating prosperity invoke the energy of Saraswati by suggesting improvement in our thinking, and envisioning higher goals for ourselves, achievable through affirmations. Ernest Holmes, founder of the Church of Religious Science, advocated the creation of new kinds of thinking about our lives and divinity. His church and the Unity Church honor and invoke the untapped powers of the mind through affirmations that the East would invoke as Saraswati. So although we may not be readily familiar with Saraswati here in the West, in some sense we already know her.

In our lives, she empowers anything involving the mind. To gain knowledge and insights concerning your every worldly pursuit, literally *anything* you do, from playwriting to woodworking, from astronomy to running a greenhouse, from creating an ad campaign to working with troubled youth, the help of Saraswati can be sought. To gain a good education for yourself or your children, the mantras of Saraswati are waiting to be chanted. To advance your understanding of the great spiritual questions, Saraswati mantras should be chanted and specific spiritual disciplines undertaken.

The power of Saraswati is illustrated here through a story that shows her involvement in the very creation of the universe.

Saraswati and the Creation of the Universe

In a realm beyond the laws of physics, beyond the minds of humans, beyond the ken of any save the most highly advanced spiritual adept, lies a reality completely different from the one we inhabit. There, a divine being, actually the *essence* of "Being," called Narayana, sleeps. Narayana exists in a realm governed by another type of mental activity altogether different from that in which we currently live. In fact, from Narayana's perspective, *this* universe, the realm *we* call home, does not exist at all. The galaxies are not even a cosmic conjecture. Sentient beings are far from consideration. But as Narayana slumbers, this four-armed androgynous being prepares to create our universe. By his very dreams, he generates the stuff of our universe, where we will be players in a divine drama acted out over billions of years.

As this particular dream opens, a lotus flower blossoms from Narayana's navel, and starts to grow. It grows and morphs until it resembles an egg in the middle of a flower from which ultimately hatches a four-faced masculine being called Brahma. Brahma represents Mind, and within him—that is, within primordial mind, or consciousness—stirs an overwhelming urge to create and multiply. Just as Narayana represents Being, Brahma is Mind. Within him, now, the Desire to propagate appears. From Mind comes Desire.

But before Brahma can do anything about his desire, two demons emerge from the ear of the sleeping Narayana. Spying Brahma, who has only half emerged from out of his birth lotus, the demons gleefully decide to exhibit the dark side of their nature. Brahma is fully conscious of his vulnerable position. He knows that something terrible may happen to him at any moment, and he yells to the sleeping Narayana to awaken and protect him. For a second, nothing at all happens and Brahma watches, horror-stricken, as the demons start to make their way over to where he rests in the flower at Narayana's navel.

But just then, a large radiant feminine figure arises out of the form of Narayana. Although he still slumbers, the feminine figure seems to come directly from Narayana's dormant body. Observing Brahma and the encroaching demons, she speaks. "Well, what have we here!"

"Help, help," cries Brahma. "I am threatened by those two evil figures even before I am completely formed. Please, wake up Narayana so that I can be saved."

The radiant feminine figure turns to the demons, who have now halted in their tracks. Briefly contemplating the situation, she muses, "I see."

"Oh, Great Mother," one of the demons speaks quickly, "we mean nothing, really."

"Oh, yes they do," gushes Brahma. "They mean me great harm, and I beg protection."

"I understand what is going on here," says the feminine figure to the demons. "I must protect this blossoming one from you two."

"We will make no harm," the demons instantly reply. "Just send us far, far away. You wouldn't kill us when we haven't actually done anything, would you?"

"Destroy them quickly," Brahma pleads, "before they attack even you."

Considering a moment, the feminine figure decides: "The sleeping Narayana has created you all. His dream will be the stuff of a new universe and there you shall all contend with one another in due course of time. For now, I command that when the universe has completed its first, etheric phase of creation, you demons shall go to the farthest reaches of that place. It will take you a long time to come back to the center of things. Meanwhile, I offer shelter and protection to you, Brahma, while you finish your act of creation."

As the demons mutter to themselves, Brahma supplicates the feminine figure with joined palms. "Great Mother, who are you? I must know the name of my savior and benefactor."

She replies, "I am the spouse of he who slumbers. I am his feminine self, his energy, his wisdom, and all power that he manifests in any form whatsoever. I am called Lakshmi. As I am to Narayana whose dream this is, I shall also be *your* power and all energy and power of this creation of yours. For you, I shall manifest as Saraswati, she who is self-contained, self-aware, and with full knowledge of that which you will create. I shall be your divine speech that you will use to create anything and everything. As your feminine aspect, Saraswati, I give you the power to create. "

Brahma found that while Lakshmi was speaking, he continued to grow and emerged from the lotus. Now that he was finally free from the flower, he beheld a different radiant feminine form. At his side, Saraswati, the embodiment of Divine Speech, looked at him with eyes that contained infinity and melted into him from head to toe. Brahma smiled. He remembered the desire he had only begun to experience when the demons appeared and disturbed his thoughts. He closed his eyes and hummed a vibrant, reverberating tone. The note hung in the blackness for a second, and then sprouted into a bubble that grew and grew, becoming larger and larger in no time at all.

At that precise moment, a ball of light emerged from the form of the sleeping Narayana. It entered the bubble and shattered into millions of sparks of light. Some pieces were bigger than others, but the majority of the multitude of splinters of light were about the same size. They would be the souls, the various forms of atman that would become the people of the new universe that was, even now, in the process of becoming.

Enjoying what she'd set in motion, the now disembodied Lakshmi spoke for the final time. "He who has made this cosmos through you is now playing in it. I shall also appear at the proper time, and you, too, will take part in this great play. As the Mind of the cosmos, you will be like the Grandfather who knows and understands all. Saraswati, your feminine counterpart, shall bless sincere seekers with wisdom and power. She shall be the pinnacle of wisdom and knowledge to whom all who love knowledge, will aspire." And with that the echo of her words faded away.

With glowing anticipation and a sense of awe, Brahma found that he could, miraculously, pierce and enter the bubble of his creation. And this he did. The expanding universe, with its concepts of time, distance, and space, had begun. Immediately, Brahma could understand why Narayana had entered his own dream. It was fun.

Just as Narayana is Being and Brahma is Mind, the great feminine energy Saraswati is Brahma's shakti, his power. She "speaks" a great idea through his mental conception and the cosmos is born. Creatures of every form and description come into existence, and the play of the universe unfolds. In this story, as divine speech, she is not unlike the power contained in the opening phrase of the Gospel of John, "In the beginning was the word," or God's divine command in Genesis: "Let there be light."

Divine Speech

For a long time, although other Eastern goddesses have gained some familiarity in the West, Saraswati has been kept under wraps. Perhaps this is because her power to reveal mysteries is so great.

Saraswati, in her manifestation as Divine Speech, represents a route, through mantra, to grasping the underlying spiritual laws of the universe and through them the attainment of personal spiritual and material power. Often referred to simply as Vach (goddess of all speech in the primordial sense, both divine and mundane), she is the primordial word used in spiritual formulas and great ceremonial observances. She is also the First Cause and the ineffable "name" of the Kabbalists. She is the power, mistress, and constructor of mantra through the phenomenon of mystical, subtle speech.

Speech is the enabler of the mind. Desires may come from the mind but they are made manifest by spoken or subtle speech. The Gayatri Mantra is considered to be the most powerful general application of divine speech, and Saraswati is said to be this mantra's essence through the syllable "Om." Om, as you may know, is the syllable or seed sound that activates the *Ajna* chakra at the brow center, which in turn activates the principle of mind.

In the structure of the creative power of sound, Nada, as Saraswati, is the primordial sound vibration emanating from the kundalini at the base of the spine, parallelling the creation of the universe. As Upamshu, she is the spoken word. She manifests as Pashyanti, or intuitive speech, when emanating from the *Swadisthana* (second) chakra. As Para, or unmanifested speech, Saraswati springs from the *Anahata* chakra at the heart center, and extends through the brow center. Thus, her power as sound is contained within us at every level of our being and spiritual development.

This Para manifestation is part of the mystical power of the great Tibetan mantra: "Om Mani Padme Hum." Pulling the energy from base to brow, mystical speech as Saraswati manifests both the universe and our place in it, through interaction between the kundalini and the chakras.

The relationship of sound to the creation of the universe is found in different scriptures originating in India. Sir John Woodroffe's *Garland of Letters* is a translation of one of the earliest recorded scriptures in all of mankind. Called the *Sata-patha Brahmana* (VI 1-1-8), it is reputed to have been part of an oral tradition in India for six to eight thousand years. It states, "In the beginning was God with power through speech. God said, 'May I be many . . . May I be propagated. And by his will expressed through subtle speech, he united himself with that speech and became pregnant. . . .'" It sounds amazingly like the Gospel of John, "In the beginning was the word, and the word was with God and the word was God."

Saraswati in Scriptural References

Not only is Saraswati the power of divine speech, she is also knowledge. In this context, Brahma is the source of all knowledge and Saraswati is knowledge itself.

Saraswati is generally pictured dressed in a white sari, unadorned; although all of creation comes into being because of her, worldly possessions are of only passing interest to her. Portrayed as having dark skin and eyes and a crescent moon in her forehead, she will have either two or four hands. Sitting on a lotus (the seat of kundalini at the base of the spine), she holds a lute (symbolic of music and the arts), a book (knowledge), rosary or *mala* (spiritual disciplines), and a hook, indicating her power to move us to the right part of the path. In some depictions she may hold a spear, showing that her mantras can have applications in the art of war, and the ceremonial bell used in Vedic religious ceremonies.

It is in *The Brahmanas* that Saraswati is first referred to as the Mother of the Vedas and the essence of the Gayatri Mantra. She is described as "The form of all that is conscious. The origin, knowledge, and perception of reality. The instigator of intellect, the ultimate goal of the yogi."

In the *Rig Veda* (V 125-5) we find references to the power she brings to those who use her mantras and perform her ceremonies: "I (Saraswati-Vach) make him who I love formidable. . . . One a Brahmana, one a rishi, one a sage. By Sacrifice (mantra) they follow the path of Vach (divine speech) and found Her entered into them."

All of these ancient references to power embodied in the human form are still applicable and functioning for you and me today. The Saraswati principle governs all spiritual pursuits, according to the ancient scriptures. Spiritual teachers and gurus (those who dispel the darkness of ignorance) transmit the power of mantra through the Saraswati principle. Followers of the path of Intellectual Understanding and Power of the Mind are similarly governed by this principle.

Gayatri, Mother of the Vedas: Giver of the Gayatri Mantra

An aspect of Saraswati that is less well known is her role as Gayatri Devi (*devi,* from which the English word *divine* is derived, means goddess), told in the *Matsya Purana* and other Puranic sources. Here is the tale of the appearance of Gayatri, who will be proclaimed Mother of the Vedas, the world's oldest scriptures, and will give the great Gayatri Mantra to Sage Vishwamitra in a future epoch. Vishwamitra, whose story is told in *Healing Mantras,* is known as the Seer of the Gayatri Mantra.

Several millennia after the etheric universe was created, with all its stars and galaxies, Brahma noticed that when certain rituals, particularly fire ceremonies, were performed in concert with certain astrological events, various life activities could be optimized for the best possible results. Whether planning a trip around the cosmos or warding off negative forces, performing the fire rituals in accordance with the stars seemed to have a positive bearing. So, when Brahma decided that he would sponsor a fire ceremony to solidify his position as "Grandfather" (the name all called him, honoring him as the mental cause of the cosmos in which he now played a role), he consulted with priests to calculate the movement of heavenly forces. The priests identified for Brahma a five-hour window during which conditions would be just right, and Brahma sent out invitations to all the gods and goddesses to attend his ceremony.

When the day arrived, he left his abode a bit early with a word to his spouse, Saraswati, that she must arrive on time to ensure that the most favorable hours not be missed. Leaving her to finish her preparations, Brahma took off for the site of the ceremony.

Taking note of the many shiny pots of gold and silver holding etheric flowers of every color and size, Brahma addressed the priests scurrying about. "What a beautiful setting you have created!" Incense of the most pleasing fragrance wafted through the area, providing an elegant air to the surroundings. Brilliant cloths upon which people would sit were spread everywhere. All was festive and in every way inviting.

"We saw to every detail, Grandfather," replied one of the priests. "It isn't every day that we are presented with such an honor and such an opportunity."

"Well, you have certainly made everything perfect. I cannot imagine a better setting for our ceremony." But Brahma was concerned because Saraswati had not yet arrived. Nervously, he asked one of the priests to go and urge Saraswati to hurry; the ideal astrological moment for beginning the ceremony was fast approaching. Nodding, the priest rushed off and soon arrived at the home of Brahma and Saraswati.

Poking his head inside the open doorway, the priest spoke with some nervousness. "Uh, Mother Saraswati, the moment for the ritual is getting ever closer and Grandfather requests your presence."

From another room, Saraswati replied unseen. "Oh, there is plenty of time. I have not yet finished dressing, and I still have a few things to do. I will be there presently."

The priest returned to Brahma with Saraswati's answer. Not at all satisfied, Brahma motioned to Indra, chief of the celestials, to come over to where he sat.

"What is it, Grandfather?" Indra asked.

"Saraswati is holding me up. The best moment for the beginning of the ceremony is coming quickly and still she is not here. I must have a wife beside me for the best possible outcome. Therefore, I ask you to find me a stand-in wife. Go quickly and return with someone."

Indra was quietly astonished, but no one refused Brahma. So he headed out to the verdant countryside, where he soon came upon a beautiful milkmaid named Gayatri who was just finishing up her chores. Striding toward her, Indra began to speak even before he had quite arrived. "Come, Grandfather requests your presence at his great ceremony. You must come with me now."

"You must have me confused with someone else, noble sir," said Gayatri. "I have never been introduced to Grandfather and am not anyone of importance."

"You are now, and there is no mistake." Indra grabbed her hand and began pulling her off toward the place where the ritual was being held.

Even as she stumbled along after him, Gayatri spoke. "Why should I be so quickly invited and dragged to this great ceremony for someone I have never even met?"

"You are to wed Brahma himself so that his ceremony goes well."

Gayatri dug her sandals into the ground and the startled Indra nearly fell over as he was suddenly forced to stop. "Brahma already has a wife, the exalted Saraswati. He does not need another, particularly a humble one such as myself."

"You have been selected because Saraswati has not arrived in a timely fashion. The optimum astrological time is just arriving and still she is not there. The stars will not sit and wait and the ceremony must begin shortly. Now come quickly and do not resist since Grandfather himself has ordered this."

Gayatri relented and once again they moved forward until they arrived at the gala setting for the ceremony.

Brahma, spying them, broke out in a smile. "Indra, you have done well. Come, beautiful one, we will have the very shortest of marriage vows and then commence the grand fire ceremony."

One of the priests hustled over to the two and with rapid phrases a brief wedding ceremony was performed in just under ten minutes. "Three days or ten minutes, what's the difference how long the marriage ceremony is." Brahma shrugged. "We are ready for the fire ritual." Taking his new bride by her elbow, he led her over to the place where she, as Brahma's wife, would sit.

But just as the ritual was getting under way, Saraswati arrived in full ceremonial attire. Her eyes could not believe what they saw and her voice quavered between outrage and deep injury. "I see it, but it cannot be true. Who is this who sits at your side, husband?"

"Since you could not tear yourself away from your dressing table, and the moment for beginning the ceremony was close, I asked Indra to find me a second wife who would sit with me." Brahma was the very picture of reason.

"And have the two of you married?" asked Saraswati.

"Oh yes, it was done most expeditiously," replied Brahma. "Come, sit beside me here." He motioned to a place slightly behind him opposite Gayatri.

"I think not." Saraswati's eyes seemed to glow ominously and Brahma instantly knew what was behind them. "You have some sinful intention to humiliate me? Have you no shame? Has lust so gripped you that you have stooped to this?" Saraswati's voice seemed to become more powerful without increasing in volume.

Vishnu, who was destined to become the tireless worker for the redemption of souls and sentient beings everywhere, tried to intervene. "O, Mistress of Divine Speech itself, no one sought to insult you. Only the time for the ceremony was on anyone's mind."

"You defend him?" Saraswati was scathing.

Now Shiva spoke. Only Brahma's formal invitation could have roused him from his meditation to attend the fire ritual. He now felt obliged to support his host. "You know well, Saraswati, that both members of a divine union are party to any result. You were not here and were asked to hurry but would not comply. Some responsibility in this matter is yours, whether or not that idea is pleasing to you."

"You also defend this traitorous act?"

"O, fair one," soothed Brahma, "forgive this seeming indiscretion. I shall never again trouble you in any way. Come sit and let us conclude the ceremony."

Saraswati turned to Brahma with contempt. "You are called the father of sages, yet you publicly act thus? How can I show my face or call myself your wife? You have acted stupidly. You say the moment is auspicious? The planets are aligned?" asked Saraswati.

"Oh, yes!" replied Brahma.

"Good." Saraswati had suddenly become the very essence of dynamic determination. "Then my words shall be even more powerful. You may think that I am easily cast aside, but you are wrong. I declare that those celestials who have been complicit in this shameful turn of events shall suffer accordingly. To you my husband, I say this: You shall not be honored in ceremonies from this day forward. No temples shall honor you. Only one day per year shall your status even be observed. As I speak now, it becomes thus."

Then she turned to Indra. "You have found this woman. So your enemies shall also find you. You will become weak, be defeated, captured, and confined to a strange place. Although you will eventually prevail, you will need the help of a supernatural drink, herbs, and other celestials to eventually win the day. Your legend as capable of defeating anything without aid will come to an end. Further, a time will come when you are so completely humiliated in battle that only a woman will be able to save you."

Then her attention shifted to Vishnu. "Your defense of his action cannot be washed away. You, more than all the others here, know the sanctity of love. When the world evolves to its physical state, your wife shall come in beauty, adoration, power, and fidelity. Yet she shall be taken from you and you shall be forced to wander in strange lands in search of her. Later, you shall be humbled by having to take care of cows, living in a simple manner in the remote countryside. You shall do this more than once. In one earthly incarnation, your beloved one shall not accompany you into human form, and you will be forced to enjoy her only in the contemplative state."

Lastly she turned her uncomfortable gaze upon Shiva. "As for you, who thinks himself ever wrapped within himself, you shall lose your manhood.* Yes, you, too, shall take a wife, cherish her, love her with great abandon, only to lose her by her own hand."

Finished with them, Saraswati turned and strode away. Some of the women who had attended the ceremony followed her for a few paces but then stopped and went back. Saraswati had a few choice words for them as well, and continued on her way.

In due course of time, all of the words of the divine Saraswati came to pass. Indra was cursed by Durvasas (Chapter 5) and became weak. When the demon Vrtas, he with no head or foot, threatened all, only the help of Vishnu, the Soma drink, and a

---

*A slang expression for celibacy, wherein supposedly all semen is retained within and transmuted into spiritual energy. She is saying that he will engage in sexual practices and lose some of his semen.

special herbal armband could help Indra prevail against the dreadful enemy. Finally, demon Mahi Asura would defeat him and send him and the other celestials into hiding, only to be saved by a woman. But that, as they say, is another story . . . (found here in Chapter 7).

Vishnu, as we will see, did indeed meet Lakshmi when the ocean of consciousness was churned, as we shall see in Chapter 5. When Vishnu incarnated on Earth as Rama, Lakshmi incarnated with him as Sita and was kidnapped by the demon Ravana. Rama was forced by court intrigue to wander in the forests for fourteen years, before eventually being reunited with Sita. When Vishnu came again to the earth as Krishna, he lived his boyhood years as a cowherd, fulfilling the words of Saraswati. And when he came again as the Buddha, Lakshmi did not come to earth with him but stayed in the etheric realm as Tara, the Great Mother.

Nor could Shiva escape the utterances of Saraswati. The rest of her words also came to pass, as we shall see in Chapter 3.

After some time, Saraswati and Gayatri met in the forest. Rather than exchange glances of hostility and mutual mistrust, they laughed and talked as intimate friends. Finally, Saraswati said, "You have done well, O my own emanation. From this time forward, householders and monks alike will chant your mantra to attain enlightenment. Through you I shall create scripture and writing. Spiritual science shall be recorded and passed from generation to generation. In my present form, I will be revered by sages and recluses of all kinds. But through you, every householder, both male and female, shall strive for the Supreme Truth. Now, for a time, let us join as one, as you are part of me and I of you." With that the two women merged.

All of this was part of the grand design of Narayana to quicken the evolving nature of the universe. After all, it was his dream, so he could do whatever he wanted.

Other Names and Qualities Ascribed to Saraswati

Because of her broad application of powers and attributes, Saraswati has collected many references and qualities. She is also called:

- Bharati in her manifestation as Eloquence
- Maha Vidya as Transcendental Knowledge
- Vach as Speech, in every aspect
- Maha Vani as the Transcendental Word
- Arya as Noble One
- Brahmi as Power of Immense Being. As Brahma's power, Saraswati inhabits Brahma entirely. Thus, if his being is as immense as the universe, she as his power is similarly a power as immense as the universe.
- Kama Dhenu as the Wish-Fulfilling Cow. Brahma Rishis and other great sages are said to be able to fulfill desires by merely thinking them so. Since the cow is a symbol of plenty in India, providing milk, butter, yogurt, and dung, which can be used as fuel, this same symbol is used to represent the munificence of spiritual abilities available to the great sages.
- Bhija Garbha as Seed of the Word
- Dhameshwari as Diversity of Wealth

Finally, Saraswati is associated with music in all its aspects and forms. If you compose songs, write musical scores, teach music, are a musician or singer or musical performer of any kind, Saraswati is the feminine archetype you should invoke.

Foundation Mantra of Saraswati

Who among us does not wish to gather knowledge and wisdom? If you are interested in science or medicine, you would probably like a deeper understanding of the laws of physics and chemistry, or have keen insights that can help you in research. If business, banking, or economics is your interest, a greater understanding of the interplay of forces that rule local commerce or the global economy would be of enormous benefit. Parents want their children to do well in school, so that their future will be ensured through knowledge that will enable them to have successful careers. A thirst for true spiritual knowledge drives many seekers. For all of these intelligence-related activities, Saraswati holds keys that unlock mysteries both mundane and spiritual.

A woman in New England whom I'll call Jody was concerned for her son in school. He was doing adequate but uninspired work in his sixth-grade class. Concerned about his study habits, lackluster results from halfhearted efforts, she e-mailed me asking if there was a mantra that could help. I suggested that she chant the foundation Saraswati mantra for good results from education, which has been used by the faithful in Asia for centuries.

1. Om Eim Saraswatyei Swaha
[Om I'm Sah-rah-swaht-yea Swaha-hah]
"Om and salutations to the feminine Saraswati principle."

Eagerly, Jody began a discipline on her son's behalf. It is axiomatic in Indian spiritual circles that parents have both a right and a duty to chant mantras on behalf of their children. If a child becomes ill, the parents will chant mantras for regaining health. If the child becomes unruly and difficult to manage for either parents or teachers, there are other mantras that can be chanted, and so forth. For educational issues, the first refuge is the Saraswati mantra given above.

After six weeks, I received another e-mail from Jody brimming with gratitude for the mantra and the results it had brought. Her son was now doing "straight A" work in school. Her gratitude was misplaced. She, herself, had done all the work. Her diligent practice with this great mantra had yielded the fruit of positive results, just as it has for centuries. I was merely a store clerk pointing to the right shelf for the goods she desired.

This Saraswati mantra is also excellent for use by musicians. I knew a composer, a guitar player, who wrote wonderful music and lyrics after completing a forty-day period of reciting this mantra for twenty minutes, morning and evening. For the task of infusing his mind with musical inspiration, the Saraswati mantra given above worked wonderfully. When I last saw him, he had not achieved the fame and fortune he desired, but for that he would have benefited from working with mantras pertaining to Lakshmi, described in an upcoming chapter.

Other Saraswati Mantra Applications

Philosophy, Mysticism, and Such

For those engaged in the study of philosophy, mysticism, and similar pursuits, the following mantra begins the process of building capacity in the brain to hold and consider great ideas. This stirs and strengthens both intelligence and intellect. The mantra describes Saraswati as the power behind the intelligence of the universe itself.

2. Om Brahma Jnanayei Namaha

[Om Brah-mah Jnah-nah-yea Nahm-ah-hah]

"Om and salutations to the power of that self-aware intelligence that pervades the universe."

Physics, Chemistry, Astronomy, and Such

For those studying physics, various kinds of chemistry, astronomy, and the like, the following mantra is efficacious. It describes Saraswati as the power behind great knowledge and its apprehension.

3. Om Maha Vidyayei Namaha

[Om Mah-hah Vid-yah-yea Nahm-ah-hah]

"Om and salutations to the power behind and producing great knowledge."

Religion

For those who delve into the ideas and texts of religion, trying to unravel the deeper meaning of scripture from any religion or culture, this somewhat longer mantra conditions the higher faculties of the mind to open to more penetrating insight. It proclaims that the energy of that understanding is actively at work within, and by this proclamation, makes it so.

4. Vedanam Matram Pasya Matstham, Devim Saraswati

[Veh-dah-nam Mah-trahm Pahs-yah Maht-sthahm Deh-veem Sah-rah-swah-tee]

"Behold, Saraswati, Mother of the Vedas resides in me."

Maha Vidya Mantra: Queen of Knowledge Mantra

This mantra is said to contain and disclose every kind of esoteric knowledge. I know a Christian minister who said this mantra for just a few weeks before reporting that she felt a strong and strange energy in her head. Thereafter, although her commitment to Jesus only gained strength, her whole life path changed. I watched in appreciation and wonder as her search for the Holy Spirit led her in a new direction. I am certain she will find what she seeks.

> **5. Eim Hrim Srim Klim Sauh Klim Hrim Eim Blum Strim Nilatari Saraswati**
> **Dram Drim Klim Blum Sah**
> **Eim Hrim Srim Klim Sauh Sauh Hrim Swaha**
> [I'm Hreem Shreem Kleem Saw Kleem Hreem I'm Bloom
> Streem Nee-lah-tah-ree Sah-rah-swah-tee
> Drahm Dreem Kleem Bloom Saw
> I'm Hreem Shreem Kleem Saw Saw Hreem Swah-hah]
> This "freight train" mantra is a succession of seed sounds and is therefore essentially untranslatable. Faithful repetition of this mantra will, over time, transform the sayer into a person of great spiritual knowledge.

Tibetans Also Propitiate Saraswati

For them, she is the spouse and power of the Bodhisattva of Wisdom, Manjushri. Holding the sword of discriminating wisdom, he is able to cut through illusion and appearance and arrive at the essential, underlying, and fundamental truth of anything. Here is his mantra.

> **6. Om Ara Pat Sa Na, Dhih Dhih Dhih**
> [Om Ah Rah Paht Sah Nah Dhee Dhee Dhee]
> "Salutations to He who is realized in the heart through the great syllable Dhi."

Gayatri Mantra: Long and Short Forms

Among all the millions of mantras recorded and stored in Far Eastern archives, the Gayatri Mantra is uniformly called the essence of all mantras. Here's why.

Similar in view to Dante's vision of Paradiso in the *Divine Comedy*, the Eastern mystical philosophy holds that the universe contains seven nether spheres of darkness and seven luminous layers of light—as above, so below. Each realm has a single vibration that summarizes its essence. Because of the way it is constructed, the Gayatri Mantra is able to bring into our subtle body the energy of each of the upper luminous *lokas*, or levels, of the universe via a single vibration.

The individual syllables of the Gayatri Mantra contain an energy seed for each of these seven planes of light. Because it contains the seeds for those realms, chanting the Gayatri Mantra builds an inner attunement with each of them. As each portion of the mantra is chanted—Bhur, Bhuvaha, Swaha, et cetera—we invoke a tiny amount of spiritual energy from that particular celestial plane into the subtle body through the action of the mantra on the chakras. Adding "Om" in front of each of these syllables ties the energy vibration to the conscious mind so that we have a mental connection to the realms as well as an energy connection.

Over time and many repetitions, each chakra becomes tuned to the energy of each of the upper luminous spheres. The ultimate result is that the entire subtle body becomes attuned with all the planes of light. We become a small microcosm of energy for the upper planes of light in the universe. Contemplating this idea gives new meaning to the idea that we are "created in the image of God."

It is one thing to be created in the image of God, it is quite another to be able to manifest that image through spiritual practices such as the Gayatri Mantra. Sustained practice of this mantra over a long period of time can produce a form of enlightenment called *Sahaja Samadhi*. This state, sometimes referred to as the natural enlightened state, enables one to live his or her daily life while in an enlightened state. Completely transparent to those surrounding such a person, the great gurus and avatars are said to be in Sahaja Samadhi even as they live among their students and followers who have no idea that their teacher, awake or asleep, or involved in daily activities, never leaves the enlightened state.

The power this mantra produces in us makes it easier to understand why many sects of Hinduism that conflict with one another on doctrinal issues practice this mantra with no disagreement among them on its efficacy. Similarly, certain Buddhist sects, such as those in Sri Lanka, also teach and practice this mantra. Sustained practice can even produce communion with beings that dwell on higher planes. I have had dream-encounters with teachers in other realms that I attribute to my extensive work with this mantra since 1974.

In daily life, faithful repetition of this mantra brings spiritual light into the physical body so that diseases are less frequent and are milder when they do occur. The prana becomes energized producing energy, inspiration, and a form of vibrational protection called *kavacha*. To those who see such things, the aura becomes bright.

There are two forms of this master mantra that I refer to simply as the long and short forms. The long form is:

7. **Om Bhur Om Bhuvaha Om Swaha**
   Om Maha Om Janaha Om Tapaha Om Satyam

Om Tat Savitur Varenyam
Bhargo Devasya Dhimahi
Dhiyo Yonaha Prachodayat
[Om Boor Om Boo-vah-hah Om Swah-ha
Om Mah-ha Om Jah-nah-ha Om Saht-yahm
Om Taht Sah-vee-toor Vah-rein-yum
Bhahr-goh Dei-vahs-yah Dhee-mah-hee
Dhee-yoh Yoh-nah-hah Prah-choh-dah-yaht]
"O Self-Effulgent light that has given birth
to all the lokas [spheres of consciousness]
who is worthy of worship and appears
through the orbit of the Sun, illumine our
intellect."

Spiritual Planes Represented (encapsulated)

Om Bhur	Earth plane	(1st chakra)
Om Bhuvaha	Atmospheric plane	(2nd chakra)
Om Swaha	Solar region	(3rd chakra)
Om Maha	First spiritual region beyond the sun:	
	Heart vibration	(4th chakra)
Om Janaha	Second spiritual region beyond the sun:	
	Power of the divine spiritual word	(5th chakra)
Om Tapaha	Third spiritual region beyond the sun:	
	Sphere of the progenitors.	
	Realm of the highest spiritual	
	understanding while still identified with	
	individual existence.	(6th chakra)
Om Satyam	The abode of supreme truth:	
	Absorption into the supreme	(7th chakra)
Om Tat Savitur Varenyam	That realm of truth which is	
	beyond human comprehension	

| Bhargo Devasya Dhimahi | In that place where all the celestials of all the spheres have . . . |
| Dhiyo Yonaha Prachodayat | . . . received enlightenment, kindly enlighten our intellect |

Short Form

For reasons I do not understand, the short form of the mantra is much more commonly practiced in the Far East than the long form. I have repeatedly asked Eastern spiritual teachers why this is so, but I have never received a satisfactory answer. Here is the short form of the Gayatri Mantra.

Om Bhur Bhuvaha Swaha
Om Tat Savitur Varenyam
Bhargo Devasya Dhimahi
Dhiyo Yonaha Prachodayat

Which Form Is Best to Use

I was initiated into the practice of the Gayatri Mantra in 1974, and was given the long form at that time. I did not even know that a short form existed. For that reason, I did not ask my initiator, Sadguru Sant Keshavadas, what the difference was between the two. Nor have I, in ensuing years, ever received a decent explanation from any other teacher, although I have asked many, many times. Therefore, I can only recommend the long form based upon my experience with it.

Finally, each of us who attains higher levels of spiritual development while on Earth performs a service for the planet and her inhabitants. Humanity has a destiny shepherded by the Great Ones. And individually, we may choose to share in The Work toward that destiny. As such choices are made, it becomes easier for humanity as a whole to advance. As such choices are made over the centuries, one day all of humanity will reach a spiritual "critical mass" and be changed forever. The Gayatri Mantra plays an important goddess-given role in the uplifting of the entire species. Whether your goals are personal or altruistic, this mantra can be of great benefit.

3

Parvati
The Power of Consciousness
and Spiritual Growth

When you are inspired to get rid of a bad habit, you have decided to grow a little. The power of consciousness moved within you, stimulated the mental power of Jnana Shakti, and you suddenly decided to give up overeating, smoking, cursing—whatever. When you actually begin that practice, Iccha Shakti, the power of will, takes over to bring the decision to completion.

When you decide that you must compose a song that will lift everyone's heart or give some important message to the listening audience, again the power of consciousness has moved within you. At first, Jnana Shakti is activated, then Kriya Shakti joins in as the creative process begins. Together, Jnana Shakti and Kriya Shakti work through you, enabling you to compose your song.

If you decide to perform more mantra practices so that you grow spiritually, the power of consciousness has again moved within you and Jnana Shakti is activated once more. Jnana Shakti plans the discipline and then Mantra Shakti takes over as your chanting starts.

What all of these examples have in common is an impulse entering the mind, coming from somewhere behind consciousness.

Mysterious, even to the yogis and sages, the power animating consciousness is a combination of all the shaktis. As the yogis know, for our consciousness to reach its highest possible attainment, the shakti, with all her powers and aspects, must ultimately move from her seat at the base of the spine, up through the spine to the crown of the head where she joins with Shiva, the masculine epitome of consciousness.

Like shakti that exists throughout the universe, Shiva (consciousness) is also really everywhere. However, for Shiva to become a kinetic consciousness, for him to achieve actual existence beyond an abstract concept, shakti must empower him. Without shakti, Shiva's consciousness is dormant, a mere blueprint of a building and not the building itself. But when Shakti provides the energy of the universe, in all of her forms, at all levels of reality, the cosmos moves from mental construct to constructed reality.

It is often said that without shakti, our body is just a corpse. But with the arrival of the soul and animation by the shakti, we begin to breathe and have existence. Not only the very power of life, this is the power that drives us to our highest possible attainment. Not just spiritually, but materially as well. It makes us desire to do well at our jobs, to wish to be good partners or good parents. It fills us with a desire to serve others, from donating our time or money to a charity to giving blood to a blood bank to volunteering to help with a community project. It powers both our dreams and desires and the means to fulfill them, providing insights and ideas for *how*.

This particular feminine force has no single name, even in the myths and stories. At different times and in different texts she is called, among other names, Uma, Sati, and Hemavati, but this incomparable feminine force is most often called Parvati.

Roles Within Roles

In the previous chapter, we saw the mythic creation of our universe begin with Narayana, a Being as incomprehensible as he is remote, sleeping in an inky void. From him, the idea of the cosmos was born. While Narayana slept, a flower opened at his navel and the creative principle, Brahma/Mind, emerged.

When Brahma was threatened by demons before he was fully born, the dazzling figure of Lakshmi appeared and saved him. Saying that she would manifest in many ways as the great feminine principle, Lakshmi disappeared, and the feminine Saraswati materialized next to Brahma as his very own shakti, or power.

Through his own feminine manifestation, Saraswati, Brahma "spoke" and the fledgling universe came into a nonphysical, etheric manifestation.

To infuse the cosmic dream with his personal divine essence, Narayana, who watched even while he slept, dispersed millions of tiny bits of his substance into the newly created universe. These sparks of light became the emerging self-conscious beings, the souls, the various manifestation of the atman that would populate this new cosmos. Some bits of this divine substance were extremely bright with almost no density and became the great rishis and sages that appear in every age. Others were of varying lesser brightness and greater density, denoting their beginning level of consciousness.

Every bit of divine material contains a capacity for linking with Narayana's essence beyond the dream, and thus can share his limitlessness, if they so choose. The working out of those choices is the action of the dream, the operation of the karma of the universe, and our karma as well.

Vishnu, as an embodiment of compassion powered by Lakshmi, will eventually pick up the reins of leadership and help us (those bits of divine substance) back to our divine source. But the stage on which this will be accomplished is built by Parvati as she forces Shiva to interact with her, and thereby makes the universe a dynamic one. From the initial vibrant tones of Saraswati's empowerment of Brahma, the mental framework for the existence of the universe was created. A fragile, etheric component of the cosmos came into existence. Much more of the universe existed in a state of potential manifestation, not yet activated.

Parvati's Story

As both consciousness in general, and as the phenomenon of individual self-consciousness, Shiva pervades the universe at every level and in everything. Shiva is usually portrayed as a solitary figure. Unconcerned with the unfolding of the universe, Shiva is intent solely upon his own consciousness and his own awareness everywhere. He is often depicted as a naked ascetic irresistibly drawn into a state of inner absorption through meditation. He is contemplating the vastness of himself, of consciousness itself.

In that activity, Shiva is really no different from any of us, because the fundamental nature of self-consciousness is to explore itself in all its fullness.

Throughout our lives, we are concerned with our desires, our wants, our needs, our enjoyments, our things, our thoughts, our families, our activities. We are ultimately completely and primarily concerned with ourselves. There is nothing wrong with this. In fact, it is the very nature of consciousness to be concerned with oneself. Who am I? What am I? Where am I going? What is my purpose? What is my relationship with other beings? And so forth. All of these questions lead naturally to a state of inner contemplation, of reflection, just like the meditative posture of Shiva.

As our story opens, Shiva, as individual consciousness, is sitting in self-contemplation, completely absorbed in universal consciousness. Parvati, the sum total of all the energy in the universe, is just being born.

Mena and Daksha knew their child was special. From the first day of her life she would gaze up at her parents, recognizing them for who and what they were: a divine couple of great consciousness and spiritual attainment. Their daily joy, she would smile coyly one minute and gurgle infectiously the next, ever engaging in pleasant infant activities that delighted her parents.

When but a few days old, the child they called Parvati began to see a strange figure in her baby dreams. Closing her eyes, within seconds she would slide into deep rhythmic breathing and enter a superconscious state wherein she saw the figure of a naked male ascetic sitting rocklike in a meditative pose. He had matted locks and bluish-colored skin; the pelt of a tiger covered only part of his slim, athletic form. For years, whenever she entered this state, the vision of this motionless young man would immediately come into her inner vision.

As a child, Parvati began to hear tales of the great ascetic Shiva, who meditated in the icy mountains to the north. Intuitively she knew that the man of these stories and the figure in her dreams were one and the same. When entering the period of her young womanhood, she realized that she desired to meet this distant and aloof mythlike person. Though he never moved, he attracted her. As she grew into full womanhood, her waking mind became filled more and more with the vision that once had appeared only in sleep and meditation. She knew that she must do something.

Well-schooled in the acts of ritual and manifestation, she uttered a prayer to the celestial Kama, who rules over the province of desire, particularly as it relates to love interests. A Hindu precursor to Cupid, Kama could send energy bolts of passion and desire into anyone, anywhere. Attracted by the power of Parvati's humble prayer, Kama appeared before her in the space of three cosmic seconds.

"Young mother of great light, I am pleased to be thus entreated by you. Though I know you not, you seem to know me. Who are you?"

"I am called Parvati, though in the future I will be known by many names," she replied. "I have asked you to come because my heart will not cease calling to the vision of one who sits in contemplation, far to the north."

"Ah, Shiva himself has his sight upon you," reckoned Kama. "Capable of seeing and being anywhere at any time, he apparently finds you pleasing in some way."

"Perhaps so. Or perhaps it is my nature that has called to him since my birth. For from the crib itself, I began to see him clearly. I feel a connection I dare not ignore." Parvati picked absently at the hem of her sari.

"Then honor it you must," replied Kama. "How can *I* help?"

"Don't play with me," Parvati gently rebuked. "It is known to all that you can infuse anything with passion. I daresay that if you desired it, stones would mate with one another."

Kama laughed good-naturedly and bent to her will. "You want me to infuse Shiva with passion for you?"

"How quickly you discern my objective," teased Parvati. "Will you?"

"Of course. It is clear that you are meant for him. I will be happy to act as divine intermediary in such an auspicious event as the union of you with Shiva. Come, we should start out immediately." Kama reached out and clasped her hand, and the two of them slipped out into the late afternoon heat to where Kama's mystical carriage awaited. They were swiftly conveyed to Mount Kailas where Shiva dwelled.

Kama led Parvati to a hilly plateau just two hundred meters from the carriage, and rising over the top of the last ridge, they could see Shiva's hut scarcely fifty meters down the ridgeline. He was seated in front of his humble abode, in the rocklike state with which Parvati was so familiar. Kama let go of Parvati's hand and proceeded down the gentle slope, speaking to her over his shoulder. "This will only take a minute, wait here until I have aroused him from his meditative slumber."

The extent of Parvati's powers was not generally known, and she preferred it that way. Seeing Kama move down the hill, she decided to darken her complexion to match Shiva's. Although some would see her as golden-skinned and others would swear that she had light skin and red lips, she now shone as a blue beauty, full of intelligence and compassion.

Kama moved stealthily to a place some fifteen meters behind Shiva, at the corner of his hut. From this vantage he directed powerful bolts of passion and desire toward the silent and unmoving figure of Shiva. After a few moments, the figure began to move.

At first gradually, then with increasing energy, the stationary Shiva emerged from the breathless state of the advanced yogi and drew in great gulps of air. Opening his eyes he swept his gaze around the horizon to find what had roused him from deep contemplation of his own universal divine nature. In less than half a second, his awareness detected Kama, and Shiva turned his handsome if somewhat stern countenance in Kama's direction. "Who is this that disturbs me?" Shiva's voice split the high altitude air like a shaft of lightning.

Kama was accustomed to being honored and appreciated. He

had not counted on Shiva's annoyance and was momentarily mute in the face of such sternness.

"Well?" Shiva said, clearly agitated.

"Ah, I am Kama, oh great yogi," he stuttered. "I have come bringing a lovely woman who desires your favor."

"So you would tempt me with carnal desire like some common animal." Shiva's anger was rising dangerously.

"I meant no harm, great sir, I—" Kama was cut off mid-sentence.

"And none shall come." With finality in his words Shiva opened his powerful third eye and emitted a bolt of energy that cut through Kama's head, reducing it to ashes. The hissing sound of Shiva's activated third eye was heard by Parvati, who jumped from her hiding place and raced down the hill.

"No, no! He was only doing what I asked." Parvati was aghast at this awful turn of events.

"And he has paid the price," said Shiva nonchalantly. He got up, strode over to where the lifeless body of Kama lay, and, reaching down, grabbed the handful of ashes that had once been Kama's head. "Now he will bother no one else." Shiva smeared Kama's ashes on his own body and returned to his seat.

Parvati slumped to the ground and tried to think of some meaningful course of action that could alter the present tragedy, while Shiva sought to return to his deep meditative state. It would not come. Shiva could not still his mind, which kept returning to the beautiful dark one who now sat just a few meters away. After a few minutes he knew it was useless. He half turned to Parvati and spoke to her with civility.

"What are you called, young woman?"

"I am Parvati. But I fear that now I may be called Parvati the Destroyer. Kama did what I asked and has paid dearly through no fault of his own."

"Knew you not that I do not like to be disturbed?" Shiva asked as gently as he could.

"I knew only that since I was a mere baby, your form in this place has ever been in my meditations and dreams. The sharpness of your temper was not revealed to me." Her eyes showed sparks of rebuke.

Shiva was unmoved. "Those who know approach me at their peril. Those who do not know should not make me responsible for their ignorance."

"But those who are meant for you should be greeted with courtesy, not hostility. Though Kama was not meant for you, I am. Thus, he should have been afforded every courtesy."

Shiva raised his eyebrows ever so slightly. This was highly unusual. People did not speak to him in this manner. To do so was to court disaster. Yet here was this—yes, attractive—young miss taking him to task with fearlessness. It was astonishing and even attractive. Shiva found he could not stop himself, and a smile appeared on his face from out of nowhere. Then mirth overcame all of his previous anger, and he melted into laughter. A hundred miles away meditating yogis stirred in their cosmic embrace as the echoing dart of Shiva's laughter startled them.

Matter-of-factly, Parvati rose and came to sit next to Shiva, arranging herself to imitate his acetic posture. "If I am to be with you, then I must also do as you do." She settled herself in.

"What are you doing?" Shiva asked.

"Being with you," Parvati replied simply.

And simple it was. The two immediately and quite naturally went into deep meditation. As Shiva returned to contemplate his innate consciousness in everything, everywhere, he found that he was no longer alone. Where before there had been only an inert consciousness, potential rather than actual, there now was an active force that made his consciousness dynamic, filled with energy and motion. This delighted him deeply. For a year he just lingered meditatively around the very concept of a dynamic consciousness pervading the entire cosmos. How different from its former state, one so inert as to be practically moribund. Parvati had become part of him in a profound way, instantly, effortlessly, powerfully.

For her part, Parvati instantly grasped and assimilated the great spiritual practices that yogis everywhere strove endlessly to achieve. Surpassing their most Herculean efforts, Parvati demonstrated to Shiva her mastery of all the hidden spiritual posture disciplines, one by one. But as she flawlessly performed each one, the heat from her efforts built throughout every quarter of creation. Finally, not only the yogis but the celestials themselves became concerned.

Selecting representatives, the celestials sent a delegation to Mount Kailas to speak with Shiva. Approaching where he and Parvati sat, eyes closed, in stonelike but dynamic silence, the head of the celestial delegation joined his palms and spoke to Shiva. "O fount of consciousness whose springs feed the universe itself, kindly harken to my humble words. Your spouse has become so quickly and powerfully adept at even the greatest spiritual practices that the substance of creation is heating to the point of discomfort and beyond. Kindly entreat her to leave off her demonstrations. We acknowledge her superiority in all these things. We respect her instantaneous attainments. We revere her presence with you here in Kailas. And we adore her compassionate nature, if she will but leave off her practices that bring increasing discomfort to the humble ones who inhabit all realms."

Opening her eyes, Parvati smiled and ceased her practices. Shiva, too, opened his eyes and took in the cringing celestial before him.

"Fear not," Shiva told him. "I am not displeased. Indeed, the mysteries of self-contemplation, all absorbing though they were, had not prepared me for the wonder of her presence. Both within and without, Parvati satisfies all needs, answers all questions, and is compassionate by nature. Is it not so, dazzling one?" He turned to Parvati.

"As you wish, so shall it be," replied Parvati artfully. "I accept the praise of you both, and am content just to be present in this place and time. Fulfilled through participation with consciousness everywhere, my nature has found its true abode. Whatever Shiva through consciousness can consider, I make it so. If it is now to be cooler that makes all happy, I blissfully comply."

Bowing to both, the celestial delegation withdrew, offering praises to consciousness and its dynamic counterpart, the Great Shakti everywhere.

Now completely enamored and accepting of Parvati, Shiva spoke to the darkly radiant figure at his side. "You have come, as you should. You have demonstrated your masterful yet compassionate nature, as is right. And you have joined me in an unexpectedly delightful way. Now I must ask, What is it you want, if anything?"

"There is nothing more fulfilling than being one with you, Lord Shiva. I ask only to be your wife." Parvati spoke simply, yet her words were elegance itself.

"Then that is what shall be," replied Shiva. "How would you like to have the formal union performed?"

"My parents have been the very model for raising a child. Therefore, I would satisfy their desires and have a traditional wedding."

"Then let us delay not one more minute," Shiva said. "We shall go immediately to your parents' home and prepare for the ceremony." And mounting Shiva's magical bull, Nandi, they sped away to the south.

Now Mena, Parvati's mother, had often heard her daughter speak of Shiva. But to hear one described as an ash-smeared figure with matted locks is quite different from actually seeing such a person. When Shiva and Parvati arrived at her home, Mena was shocked at the sight of Shiva. He looked dreadful, his tangled hair crawling with bugs. A tiger skin was wrapped loosely around his waist and draped over one shoulder. It looked as if it had never seen a river, let alone a washing tub. And what was that around his neck? My God, it was a snake! Mena fainted.

After feverish efforts to revive her, Mena eventually came around and spoke to them for the first time. "If you marry this man I will take my life by my own hand. You cannot be serious about settling down with this mangy fellow."

"Mother, long ago did you not teach me that looks can be deceiving? That I should not judge solely on the basis of appearance?"

"Yes, child, but this!" Mena broke off, unable to speak more.

"This man is meant for me and I for him. From my childhood dreams, which you know very well, to my travels to meet him, there has been no one else. Pray give up this prejudice and meet my beloved without rancor."

At these and similar sweet words Mena was placated and eventually came to meet Shiva. Observing all decorum, Shiva won her over. Parvati's father, Daksha, was another matter. He never liked Shiva. Convinced that his future son-in-law was a ne'er-do-well of the worst kind, Daksha was barely civil to him no matter how well-behaved Shiva was or how polite his speech. Because of his devotion to Parvati, Shiva let nothing of her father's bad manners concern him; he remained even-tempered and waited patiently for the day of their marriage.

Daksha could not resist Parvati's forceful insistence that the marriage ceremony be performed on a grand scale at the first astrologically beneficial moment. Thus, in just a few days, word was put forth that Parvati and Shiva were marrying and all were welcome.

When the joyous day arrived the first matter was the procession of guests, with each guest trailing either the groom or the bride according to their attachments and sentiments. While Parvati's procession was composed of the usual complement of well-wishers, friends, and families of Mena and Daksha, Shiva's procession struck fear into the hearts of all.

Grizzled sages of every sort fell in line. With dirty garments, soiled animal skins, beards and tangled hair of every color and length, the sages were only the beginning. Next came goblins and foul figures, terrible to behold, from the lower realms of existence. With bulging eyes, long hideous tongues, and grins filled with memories of terrible deeds, the only thing all of these frightening creatures had in common was their utter devotion to Lord Shiva. For his sake, on this wonderful day of union, all were on their absolutely best behavior.

Daksha was completely disgusted at the unsavory procession of Shiva's entourage. It was insulting, he thought, that such creatures were free to come to his daughter's wedding. Daksha knew that Shiva could have mandated that "only those who will not frighten others are welcome at my wedding." Those devoted to Shiva would have honored his request, and Daksha and Mena's guests would not have arrived only to faint out of fear. No, this Shiva fellow had gone way too far, thought Daksha. But Daksha did not understand that self-awareness is a state that knows no difference among good and evil, high and low, saintlike or devilish.

Shiva knew that each kind of being and each individual creature has its unique nature. "You cannot expect the butterfly to have the same sensibilities as the bumblebee," he would say. "Nor the deer the same as the tiger. Yet all may find repose and comfort within my unprejudiced conscious embrace. So long as each creature is sincere within the limits of its nature, I am completely satisfied." Because Shiva treats all who propitiate him with total equality, beings from every realm, both low and high, chant his mantras and sing his praises.

After the procession and marriage vows were exchanged, the postwedding festivities commenced. With a last comment from Shiva to his invited guests to behave themselves, Shiva and Parvati escaped back to Mount Kailas.

Now that the formalities were disposed of, Shiva could at last reflect within himself and acknowledge the depth and breadth of desire he possessed for Parvati. Kama had done his work well. And although Shiva was the very model of restraint in every way, nonetheless, the fire of passionate desire burned strong and deep. Nor was Parvati any less desirous of passionate union. So, with great joy and careless lack of further restraint, they engaged in lovemaking to the fullest extent of their capacities. Their rapturous embrace lasted long, with its vibrations cascading down Mount Kailas, into the celestial realms, into the lower depths, and out into the far reaches of space and time.

After a while, however, the celestials began to get nervous. What if the fire of their union should become so intense that the universe began to burn, destroying everything? What if the intensity of their joy should shatter the concept of time so that no being who lived by the principle of duration could survive? In their minds, the very *ideas* of time and space were threatened by the union of Shiva and Parvati. It was decided that the two should be interrupted. Only by ceasing their lovemaking could the universe be preserved, or so the celestials thought.

Creeping up on the unsuspecting couple, a delegation of celestials commenced to make such a racket of mock celebration that Shiva and Parvati were, indeed, momentarily startled from their deep mystical embrace. Emerging from their ecstatic union, something completely unforeseen occurred. A tiny drop, a mixture of semen and feminine fluid, escaped and fell to the ground. So powerful was this drop that the etheric universe could not contain the tiny potent mixture, and it slipped through a crack in the time-space continuum, plunging into realms that were yet to be created. Saraswati's words had come to pass, as she knew they would.

On and on the drop fell until it entered the future potential universe where the Earth would be created. In their potential states, not yet actualized in tangible existence, the various elements sought to contain and stop the drop. But the element of air could not contain the drop without becoming incandescent. Fire could not contain it lest it be consumed itself, as it consumed other things. The Earth said, "I am not yet ready, I cannot contain it." But the River Ganges, knowing that the soulful prayers of millions upon millions of devotees of the divine would wash her and cool her again and again, said, "I will receive the drop." And she did, carrying the drop as it developed into a child, later to be called Subramanya. Eventually this child would be a powerful ally to souls striving for spiritual evolution while struggling on the Earth plane. In planting the seed that would become Subramanya on the threshold of the physical universe, Shiva and Parvati were complete in every way. From this day on they would humbly play out their roles as supreme masculine and feminine archetypes, consciousness and manifestation dancing together.

But now they just yawned and stretched pleasurably. "What is it?" Shiva asked the noisy well-wishers. "You have some news for me?"

Although news was not the purpose of this visit, there *was* something to report. "Please excuse this untimely interruption," begged one of the celestials. "Daksha, Parvati's father, has decided to conduct a fire ceremony. . . . A really grand observance. Unfortunately, the two of you are not invited. Even though the news is unfortunate, we all decided that you should know."

Parvati became incensed. For her father not to invite them to a large family fire ceremony was a grave insult. She was beside herself.

Shiva tried to placate her with words of reason and calm. "Dearest and most beautiful, I care not that we have not been invited. Nor should you. We are capable of having a sublime time together, alone. We need nothing and no one. Please do not be upset over something so trivial as this."

The party of celestials crept silently away. They had successfully completed their mission, but now the mountain air was becoming unsettled, as Parvati became more upset with each passing second.

"Trivial? You think my honor is trivial?" replied Parvati hotly. "It is well known that the first fire ceremony after a wedding is auspicious for the bride and groom. My father has done this to insult not only me, but you as well."

Shiva was unconcerned. "I care not what goes through your father's mind. He is not worth my time. It is my view that the only worthwhile thing he has done is to raise you. Now that you are here, he can do nothing to harm us. Let it go, divine one."

"Certain things are not to be done," Parvati insisted. "The universe runs according to firm laws. Society, too, runs according to customs and moral traditions that make it stable as well as viable. My father has violated these customs and laws most grievously." She thought for a moment and then continued. "I will go to this ceremony. It is not unseemly for family members to arrive, even uninvited, for such an auspicious event."

"That is quite true," observed Shiva, "but what do you expect to accomplish?"

"I will embarrass them for not inviting us," said Parvati simply.

"For us to be omitted from the guest list clearly shows that Daksha has no shame. You will not embarrass him in the least." Shiva spoke the truth, knowing Parvati would not be dissuaded.

"May I use your Nandi as transport? That way even though you are not present, they will know your spirit is with me." Parvati's eyes glowed with indignation.

"Of course," replied Shiva.

Shortly thereafter, Parvati departed for the south and soon arrived at her parents' home where grand preparations were under way. Greeted by friends and neighbors as an honored guest, she made her way through the gathering throngs to where her father, Daksha, was supervising arrangements. Even though he saw her, he neither went to her nor acknowledged her presence.

Parvati immediately understood that the snub was intended to be the very pinnacle of insult. Seeing this, she spoke to him in low, almost threatening tones. "Your conduct is more befitting of a demon than of a celestial. You have abandoned good judgment, common courtesy, and family obligations all in a single act. But I am not without recourse. I return the insult in the tradition of our clan and general society. I will have you as my family in this life no longer." With that she left her body, which fell over dead at his feet.

Daksha was astonished and Mena shrieked in agony. On Mount Kailas, Shiva, who had been meditating, opened his eyes in horror. Grief-stricken and enraged, he recalled Nandi with his mind, mounted the husky animal and quickly sped to the scene of Parvati's death. As Shiva arrived, two of Parvati's young women friends were trying to lift her body. Mena had fainted and Daksha's head was turned away in denial of his role in her passing.

"Leave her!" thundered Shiva. "I, myself, and no other shall bear her body." With agony in every step, Shiva walked toward Parvati's lifeless form as a rage against Daksha began to seethe inside him. Throwing Parvati's lifeless body over his shoulder, Shiva strode to where Daksha stood, his face still looking in the opposite direction from where she had fallen. Without a word, Shiva sent a blast from his third eye and reduced Daksha to ashes on the spot. Then turning away, Shiva began to wander aimlessly, still carrying Parvati's body.

Since the time Kama sent his bolts of passion, Shiva had been unable to completely withdraw into his state of total self-absorbed contemplation. Now matters were worse. His greatest joy had been taken from him. With Daksha's death his revenge was complete, but it was not at all satisfying. Filled with torment and longing for Parvati, Shiva began to wander aimlessly though the multitudinous levels of the universe.

Again the celestials had cause to worry. Because of Shiva's grief, the days were starting to vary in length. Distances could no longer be gauged with accuracy. A short trip one day would require all day the next, as the cosmos seemed to wobble precariously. Something had to be done. Seeking the highest counsel they could think of, they went to Shiva's friend Vishnu and asked his advice.

"Oh, savior supreme," began Indra the chief of the celestials, "your compassion for sentient life everywhere is known throughout all the realms. You can see now how the universe mutters to itself, not able to decide even how long should be the day and the night, or what should be the proper distance from one celestial body to another. You also must know that the cause for these conditions is the ravaging grief that holds Shiva in its grip. Please, intercede, we implore you."

Nodding, Vishnu answered, "When the sincere friend or devotee calls, and you are both, Indra, I am immediately available." Whereupon, Vishnu rose and went in search of Shiva.

It did not take Vishnu long to find Shiva, for his tears left a trail on the cosmic landscape. Vishnu kept out of sight while he observed his friend's behavior. Although he could make out no words, it was clear that Shiva was talking to Parvati, commenting as he trudged along carrying her body. Seeing this, a plan formed in Vishnu's mind. Remaining hidden, he crept up on Shiva, carrying a sharp knife. As Shiva turned in this direction or that, Vishnu would cut away a piece of Parvati's body, allowing it to fall to the ground. For many days Vishnu continued to follow Shiva, using each new opportunity to lighten his burden, bit by bit.

Finally, only a small hank of hair remained; there was nothing left of Parvati. Recognizing this as a sign, Shiva sighed, threw off the mantle of his grief, and started back to Mount Kailas. His journey took him back over ground he had aimlessly covered in his torment, and he noticed that something wondrous had happened. Wherever a piece of Parvati's body had fallen, a temple or holy place had been built. Prayerful throngs attended each one with reverence and piety. Each place had its unique qualities, customs, praises, and name for the Great Feminine.

With a lighter step and the beginnings of a smile, Shiva understood it all as a message from Parvati. Changing course, he returned to the place where he had reduced Daksha to ashes. There, Mena was living alone in sadness. Shiva entered the cottage and went directly to the place where Daksha's ashes were held in a jar. Pouring them out, he uttered the mystic *sanjivani* mantra that, when chanted by a true master, restores the dead to life. Instantly

Daksha sprang up whole from his own ashes, and Mena wept with joy. Then, together, Daksha, Mena, and Shiva performed the great fire ceremony that Daksha had planned, using the occasion to chant to the Great Feminine as an oblation to the departed Parvati. When the three-day ceremony was concluded, Shiva returned to Kailas.

But as Shiva trudged up the short path leading from the last ridge to his hut, there was Parvati waving cheerfully to him from the porch! Running the last few meters, Shiva swept Parvati up in a heartfelt embrace, and they sat down together wrapped in smiles and mutual appreciation. After lingering with each other for several hours, Parvati rose to prepare tea. "When I return," she said, "I have some questions for you."

"Whatever answers I have shall be immediately yours," Shiva replied.

Soon Parvati returned with a tray set with a steaming pot. When they had warmed themselves with several deep drafts from their cups, Parvati set hers down, joined her palms and spoke. "You who are one with consciousness everywhere are privy to every mystery in this cosmos. There are no secrets that could ever be kept from you, except you allow it. Thus, Vishnu's stealth must have been known to you, yes?"

"Of course, dearest part of me, it could not be otherwise as you know."

"And you understood my message to return Daksha to life?" Parvati continued.

"It was as clear as the breath on a cold morning." Shiva knew something was coming, but allowed himself not to see what it was.

"I have a favor before I ask my questions," said Parvati.

"I thought these were the questions," Shiva replied brightly.

"No, these are just some assurances," Parvati continued.

"What is your favor, so that I may quickly fulfill it?" Shiva asked.

"By the power of Yoga known only to one such as you, I request you also bring Kama back to life . . . only not here. Let him come back at his own place. And he need not remember what has happened, for he would only relive the pain and be unable to continue his task of inspiring beings to all kinds of passion."

"It is done this moment," replied Shiva. "Now your questions."

Parvati spoke that which had been on her mind since the beginning. "Kindly instruct me in the highest mysteries of consciousness within this creation. And please know full well that I shall test the power of whatever you teach me and then pass this knowledge on to the deserving ones. Prone as you are to slipping into cosmic introspection, I must ensure that those who show sincere piety and devoted discipline, whose lives are dedicated to knowing and serving truth, are rewarded in the ways appropriate. I pray, therefore, kindly instruct me."

"With joy and appreciation for you in every way," Shiva answered, "I shall impart all that you ask. I know that your capacity for hearing and remembering is infinite, so I shall not worry that what I have to say will take some time."

After taking another long drink of tea, Shiva gave to Parvati a set of teachings that were later written down and passed on from teacher to student. The full set of teachings is known today as the *Maha Nirvana Tantra*, or the Path of Great Power to Liberation. Through this work, many mantras of extraordinary power have been carefully recorded and explained by the eminent Sir John Woodroffe of Great Britain, who translated it under the pseudonym of Arthur Avalon.

Here are some of the mantras contained in the *Maha Nirvana Tantra* with brief explanations of the power they contain.

Brahma Mantras

Although Saraswati is the power of Brahma, it is left to Parvati to extract some of Saraswati's secrets from the consciousness of Shiva. This first mantra taught by Shiva to Parvati simply affirms that the nature of one's true consciousness in the form of an active self-aware mind is always at one with the "Mind" of the universe.

1. Sat Chid Ekam Brahma
[Saht Cheed Eh-kahm Brah-mah]

Sat	Truth
Chid	Spiritual mind stuff
Ekam	Solitary and unitary, as in, one without a second
Brahma	The "mind" inherent of all parts and manifestations of the created universe

For those who are called to experience the totality of existence through the mind, this mantra is a mine of unparalleled value. It is a mantra that very advanced teachers give to their advanced students. After some time, this mantra is expanded to contain potent "seed sounds" that greatly amplify the feminine power.

Om Eim Hrim Shrim Klim Sau Sat Chid Ekam Brahma
[Om I'm Hreem Shreem Kleem Saw Saht Cheed Eh-kahm Brah-mah]

Om	Energy to the brow center or chakra
Eim	Seed sound for the energy of Jnana Shakti ruled by Saraswati
Hrim	Seed sound for the energy of Para Shakti and of the Hrit Padma, or sacred heart
Shrim	Seed sound for the energy of Kriya Shakti ruled by Lakshmi

Klim	Seed sound of attraction that amplifies syllables around it
Sau	A kundalini shakti–activating sound also associated with the Anahata chakra, or Spiritual Heart center and its relationship to the Ajna (brow) chakra

The rest of the mantra is explained above. Serious students of spiritual advancement should alternate their practice between these two mantras, since one accents the "mind" aspect and the other emphasizes the "power of the mind" aspect. Saying the first one ten thousand times and then the second one ten thousand times will give you a taste of the power and mental horizons offered by still deeper work. If you find working with these mantras difficult, then there are other equally powerful mantras that may be better suited to you. We all have different predispositions, karmically speaking. No one path or mantra is superior to another. There is only that which is best for each of us as an individual. That and nothing more.

I know of a professional healer I'll call Penny, who practiced both of the above mantras for several months simply because she felt drawn to them. Within days of completing her own discipline, she received an assignment of significant financial worth. She also added a new technique to her skill set, with which she expects to bring in more business. Although she did not perform mantra disciplines for these purposes, it is quite true that mantra practice often brings unexpected rewards. In her case, Penny had unknowingly removed karmic circumstances that stood in her way through use of this mantra discipline.

Shakti as Shiva

Scores of mantras for various spiritual practices and tasks are introduced in chapter after chapter of the *Maha Nirvana Tantra*.

Parvati, the ideal student, prompts Shiva to reveal mystery after mystery and mantra after mantra. After several chapters, Shiva presents another powerful mantra related to Parvati herself as the sum total of energy of the potential and actualized cosmos, just as Shiva is the representation of the sum total of consciousness of the potential and actualized cosmos.

2. Hrim Shreem Klim Param Eshwari Swaha
[Hreem Shreem Kleem Pah-rahm Ehsh-wah-ree Swah-hah]

Some of the sounds have been explained above. The new ones are:

Param   Supreme
Eshwari Feminine principle (generic)
Swaha   I salute, and, I invoke

This short mantra is extraordinarily powerful. In fact, in India, the Kula sect, who are worshipers of Shiva, employ this mantra to achieve oneness with Shiva. They see no ultimate distinction between Shiva and Shakti.

Shiva as Shakti

The foundation mantra for Shiva, promulgated by the Siddha tradition, is:

3. Om Namah Shivaya
[Om Nah-mah Shee-vah-yah]
"Om and salutations. May the elements and consciousness of this creation abide in me in perfect manifestation."

In some advanced texts, this mantra is amplified by the inclusion of seed sounds to increase the power of the mantra. One such rendering uses the seed sound for Lakshmi's abundance, Shrim (Lakshmi is discussed in the next chapter), and the seed sound for attracting both abundance and the consciousness residing naturally in the elements of creation, Klim.

Twenty years ago I completed a spiritual discipline of which this was a significant part, and was given a new consulting assignment that allowed my family to move from an apartment into a house. I knew it was no accident, because events moved quickly within two weeks of my performing the discipline. Here is yet another example of something done for spiritual purposes that had a direct effect on mundane circumstances. Some spiritual teachers might say that by sweetening our material pot, so to speak, God is encouraging us to continue. Others might point to reduction of karma allowing new energy to flow into our lives. Either explanation could be true.

Om Shrim Klim Namah Shivaya
[Om Shreem Kleem Nah-ma Shee-vah-yah]
"Om and salutations. May the elements and consciousness of this creation abide in me in perfect and abundant manifestation."

Parvati's Legacy

See what Parvati has wrought. Before her appearance upon the cosmic scene, Shiva was totally absorbed in meditation, his consciousness—the consciousness of the universe, largely inert and more potential than actual. Through Kama, Parvati introduces the idea of passionate procreation and finally gains Shiva's total attention, drawing him out of his inward focus and into a fully conscious engagement with the phenomenal world. She teaches him that passionate involvement in the world has a place that is not only spiritual but also leads to a greater expression or manifestation of his potential.

To bring ideas to fruition, the energy of the Great Feminine is an absolute requirement. In this story we see that although passionate desire may be subdued (Shiva reduces Kama to ashes) it can never be eradicated (at Parvati's request, Kama is brought back to life by Shiva). Nor should it. Kama's influence is essential to the eventual manifestation of Shiva's potential, as Parvati directs and energizes its unfolding.

When Vishnu with his knife saws off pieces of Parvati, it is like the seeding of divine feminine energy in the various places that are pilgrimage spots on Earth today. Shiva learns in this way about the interrelationship between mind and matter. His passion for Parvati, combined with the energy of her material form, produces and permeates these holy places where sincere seekers may commune with and propitiate the energetic archetype, the divine feminine. Neither mind alone nor energy alone could have accomplished this. The newly enlightened Shiva brings back Daksha from the dead and then assists him in the fire ceremony. This shows Shiva is not only involved in worldly affairs, but is also involved in those activities that salute the very nature of the relationship between pure consciousness and its energized form. Finally, Parvati induces Shiva to reveal great mysteries that will produce unrivaled states of individual consciousness through mantras of supreme potency.

Subramanya, who was born of that fateful drop of divine semen and feminine fluid carried by the Ganges, was the couple's firstborn. In Vedic thought, Subramanya symbolizes the highest possible conscious attainment while still identified as an individual being. His story will appear in a future book. Later, Parvati and Shiva will create their second offspring, Ganesha. This much-beloved elephant-headed one is the symbol of unity and cosmic consciousness available to us even while we occupy a physical form.

4

Lakshmi
The Power of Abundance

Fulfilling basic needs and wants in everyday life can make things so much easier. Even the Buddha used to say that you cannot teach people how to meditate if they are starving. First you feed them, and then it becomes easy to teach people spiritual practices. Even though we may have enough food to eat and basic shelter, we all have desires and longings for items and conditions that, if satisfied, will aid every other aspect of our existence.

On any given day, particles of desire streak through the cloud chamber of our minds, leaving trails of longing that clamor for immediate fulfillment. This litany of desires for increased abundance is almost universal among us.

"I need a new car. My old one is about dead."

"I need a raise. I can barely make it on what I take home."

"I want a better job. My boss is driving me crazy."

"I need a new and bigger house. The kids need their own rooms and Mom may have to come live with us."

"I just want a lot of money. There are so many charitable causes I want to help, I need more money to help them and still provide for my family."

79

Sometimes the desires for abundance take a slightly different form.

"I'd like to be more attractive."

"I'd like a more pleasing personality."

"I'd like more friends. Everyone has moved away."

Familiar thoughts like these seem to be part of our nature. The drive to fulfill reasonable wants, to improve our surroundings with more and better "things," to improve some facet of the way we "present" ourselves to others, to enhance our enjoyment of life or guarantee future economic security appears very early in our lives.

We learn that education is a route to improving chances for good employment with its income and security perks. From childhood on, television shows us a world brimming with the joys of affluence, presented in contrast to the horrors of poverty. The choice is clear very early on: More is usually better. So it's not surprising that we have all learned how important it is to spend a significant amount of time and effort to increase the quantity and quality of our abundance. It makes things easier and enables us to help others in addition to ourselves.

The idea of abundance is not limited to money. In places around the globe where want and deprivation prevail, abundance simply means enough food to eat. Under such conditions, food for the immediate family is the first concern. If we live alone or have seen many of our friends and loved ones pass away, true wealth can be new friends and increased companionship. In this context, friends and associates are abundance. If sickness and infirmity plague our daily existence, health is abundance. Abundance is many things in addition to the financial prosperity we usually associate with it.

As part of our life, we are always making course corrections to increase those forms of abundance that are important to us. We make changes in jobs, relationships, planning strategies, investments, and other facets of our lives trying to optimize our chances for increased abundance. We usually think we know which activities will produce the results we want. However, things often do not necessarily work out as we had planned. For some people, effortless activity produces one abundant result after another. But for others, repeated attempts at fulfilling desires and accumulating abundance produce nothing but frustration and failure.

While, as we discussed earlier, an individual's karma will determine the ease or difficulty they experience in attaining certain of their desires, we also now know that we can work with universal forces to get around and eventually eliminate these limitations, if we only know what to do.

In Chapter 2 we met a fundamental feminine power called Lakshmi. She is the very epitome of abundance. According to scriptures written about her (principally, the *Shri Suktam* and *Lakshmi Tantra*), not only can she bestow abundance, she is the very source of it.

The oldest references simply refer to Lakshmi as Shri (Shree). In early Vedic hymns, Shri is she who bestows capability, power, and skillful means that manifest as beauty, luster, glory, and high rank. The later writings such as the mentioned *Lakshmi Tantra* refer to Shri as the ruling power, dominion, and majesty of kings and queens. In some texts Shri is referred to as a cushion upon which the royal ones sit. Those who are schooled in Eastern mysticism will recognize immediately that this cushion represents the kundalini shakti residing at the base of the spine in us all. In this context, to sit upon her cushion means to rest upon the power that she can and will provide, if only we know how to invoke or activate it.

There are two different myths concerning the genesis of Lakshmi in the universe. The first states that she was born of the spiritual practices, or disciplines, of ancient spiritual beings called the Prajapati.* She is said to have been a direct product of their practice of yoga and meditation.

But by far the most common myth surrounding her appearance is connected to the churning of the ocean of consciousness shortly after the birth of the cosmos itself.

The duality of the universe had already manifested through Narayana, whom we met in Chapter 2. The etheric universe came into existence and the drama of Narayana's dream began. Good and bad, positive and negative, masculine and feminine, yin and yang, centrifugal and centripetal—all the dualistic forces existed in an etheric, nonphysical state where they played out for a long time. In this etheric realm of duality, the good forces of the celestial beings constantly strove against the bad forces of the demons for overall supremacy. First one group would gain the advantage, then the other side would prevail for a time.

Both groups knew that eventually there would come a state of stasis or rest where the existence of the universe would effectively end, much like a wind-up clock that runs down and finally stops altogether. The universe, with them included as part of it, would cease to exist. Naturally, ceasing to exist was not an eventuality that either the demons or the celestials looked forward to with any pleasure. The only thing that could protect them from death at the end of the universe was a precious substance known as the Nectar of Immortality. Whoever drank this nectar would never perish.

---

*According to John Dowson, in *A Classical Dictionary of Hindu Mythology and Religion,* the Prajapati are, "Ten 'mind-born sons' of Brahma from whom mankind has descended. These ten sages are referred to as the forefathers of the human race. They are Marichi, Atri, Angiras, Pulasta, Pulaha, Kratu, Vasista, Daksha, Brigu and Narada."

Unfortunately, in the persistent battling, the nectar had been lost. The only way to retrieve the Nectar of Immortality was to churn the ocean of consciousness. This was a big job. Too big for either the forces of good or of evil to accomplish alone. Successful churning would require unprecedented cooperation. Out of their combined efforts, Lakshmi, the Goddess of Abundance, would appear and our physical universe would be born. This telling is drawn from a variety of sources, but principally from the *Vishnu Purana*.

Birth of Lakshmi

Indra looked around cautiously at the gathering of divine celestials and troublesome demons. He did not like what he saw, but there was little he could do about it. Even though he was chief of the celestials, his authority was limited, and he was now forced to go through with the hard-fought agreement that dictated coming events. He, himself, had brought the celestials to their present predicament and he was out of other options.

Some months earlier, at a gathering of celestials, Durvasas, a crusty etheric sage of irascible nature and great power, had been honored with a fragrant garland that gave him pleasure to display around his neck. Shortly after Durvasas received his garland, Indra had passed by.

"Is it not beautiful?" asked Durvasas rhetorically.

"It's all right, I guess." Indra shrugged.

Incensed that Indra was so dismissive of the beautifully composed collar of flowers, Durvasas uttered a curse whereby the power of Indra as leader of the celestials would be weakened in the etheric cosmos. Durvasas did not know, of course, that Saraswati had set all of this into motion eons ago by a few well-chosen words when Brahma had wed Gayatri.

The demons had seized this advantage and begun to wage war on the celestials, sometimes gaining an advantage. Still, neither side could prevail and both sides knew that if they did not retrieve the Nectar of Immortality, eventually all would die, even if this demise would not come to pass for thousands and thousands of years.

After a truce, Indra called a meeting of the celestials and the demons and spoke to the assembled. "If we are to be truly immortal, we must find a way to churn this ocean of consciousness. Otherwise, we will all drift endlessly in ghostly forms, ceaselessly combating one another for supremacy over a fluidic space that has neither substance nor inherent value. Churning this ocean will inevitably reveal the location of the Nectar of Immortality we all seek."

There was, of course, a catch. It was clear that only together could they retrieve the nectar. Yet if drunk by all, both the celestials and the demons would be immortal in all the worlds. This would certainly mean unending conflict between the two groups for an eternity. But there was no other way.

"I agree," said one of the demons, spitting forth his words from a twisted vile face. "Let's get on with it."

Indra continued. "First we must find a center for our churning. Our efforts will create huge forces of a centrifugal and centripetal nature. Somehow they must be contained and directed to our use. I am open to suggestions." He always thought of himself as being in charge, even when in the company of his adversaries, the demons.

"Part of my consciousness is anchored in an etheric mountain of such strength that it will not shatter from the forces you will all put forth," said Shiva. "I offer Mount Mandara as a churning stick. Further, I have asked the great savior of individual volitional awareness, my friend Vishnu, to invest a portion of himself as Kurma, the tortoise. It is upon his heroic back that the churning may rest without tearing apart the fabric of this etheric universe. Finally, I can happily announce that the serpent Vasuki has volunteered to be used as a churning rod so that you all may have some place to grasp in the churning efforts." Turning to the serpent, Shiva spoke. "You shall always be dear to me for your volunteering in this way." Vasuki nodded nervously, and prepared to fasten himself to Mount Mandara. Soon it would begin.

"Places everyone," signaled Shiva, and the entire company of demons and celestials began to move to the periphery. Vasuki dove under the top wave of the ocean to fasten his tail to Mount Mandara and then surfaced once more. Eyes glittering nervously, he nodded to Shiva. Parvati glanced at the assembly and released an infinitesimally minute portion of energy that allowed them all to commence their activity. Grasping Vasuki, the celestials and the demons began to pull his length around and around, causing Mount Mandara to rotate on its axis. The churning of the etheric ocean of consciousness had begun.

Faster and faster the celestials and the demons raced around the center point, and the ocean began to roil with the flakes of matter that would eventually become the physical universe as we know it. Around and around the center the assembly pulled on Vasuki with ever-increasing intensity and speed. Then, something completely unexpected happened. Vasuki, getting dizzier and dizzier with every round, became ill. With an eruptive cough he sent a huge projectile of poisonous substance spewing forth from his mouth. It was headed right for a large group of celestials.

Instantly moving from his neutral stance, Shiva shot across the ocean of consciousness and caught the deadly glob in his mouth. It settled into his throat where he neutralized it, even as the poison turned his throat blue. Smiling, he returned to Parvati's side knowing that hundreds of songs would be written about him in the future, praising him as the beneficent blue-throated one.

He merely said, "Go on," and the churning resumed. Parvati flicked her glance upward and the combined party of celestials and demons found that they had renewed energy and resumed their mad dash around and around the center, creating more and more building blocks of the physical universe.

Before the churning was even half-complete, wondrous and magical items began to precipitate from the ocean of consciousness. Various of the churning celestials and demons began to claim the bounty of unexpected items as they emerged from the cosmic soup. The great orb of the moon, Chandra, gloriously appeared. Not lifeless like today, this moon was full of vitality and destined to bear great rulers of humanity in a future epoch. Other precious items also arose from the whirling brew of light, consciousness, and energy.

A celestial elephant appeared that Indra immediately claimed for himself as his mount. Glaring around, he dared any of the demons or celestials to oppose him. Precious stones, a magical tree, and the manifesting power of the great Brahma Rishis, a wish-fulfilling cow, as well as other items also appeared and were claimed one by one.

Near the peak of the churning, a compact and dazzling multicolored gem appeared, of such brilliance that it caused gasps of appreciation from the whirling assembly of celestials and demons. Even though both camps desperately wanted this brightly pulsing gem, neither had any understanding of its uses or powers. By its own radiant energy, it floated over to the ever-compassionate Vishnu and melted into his chest one hand-width below the notch at his throat. Automatically, Vishnu began to speak. "This jewel, the Kaustubha Gem, has chosen me as its abode. Through its power, I can make a thing happen by speaking out loud or by speaking silently. Whatsoever I utter with dedicated purpose, it will become so. Blessed by Saraswati, this is the great wish-fulfilling gem that I will now use for protection of the pious and to safeguard the development of saintly souls. I shall allow a portion of it to reside in those who are dear to me, who aid me in my divine tasks." Finished with his explanation, Vishnu turned back to the task of churning the ocean and exerted himself mightily.

Suddenly, a shining woman of extraordinary beauty arose from the surging, swirling mists. Clad in a deep pink sari, and bedecked with gold and precious stones, she floated to the side of the celestials and alighted softly. Even though her dress and ornaments would have commanded many fortunes of extravagant kings and queens, it was not that which drew rapt attention. So strikingly radiant with both beauty and compassion was her face that all were reduced to gaping. None of them had ever seen anything like her before. She was Lakshmi, sovereign spouse (and part) of Narayana himself, regal and supreme.

For a long time, not a word was said as they all rested their troubles and cares in the soothing balm of her glance. Gone were the cares of conflict. Forgotten was any worry of the universe ceasing to be. Completely absent was any thought of the Nectar of Immortality or the churning of the ocean of consciousness or any other matter that had seemed all-important just moments ago. Only the peace-giving serenity of her glance mattered. Resting in her gaze, all were completely satisfied in every way. Finally, she cast her eyes upward and spoke only one word, "Narayana," and then lowered her eyes.

The magic moment was now over and the needs and cares of the moment returned in a rush. Indra stepped forward and, heaving out his chest, spoke loudly to the celestials and demons. "I claim this woman as my own. As chief of the celestials, I demand this right. If any among the Asura (demon) clan would oppose me, take up your weapon and stance. I am ready." No one moved. "Good," said Indra, "now come and stand beside me, O dazzling one."

Lakshmi stepped forward and spoke. Her voice was like the most pleasing music. "Narayana has sent me here to show you the Nectar of Immortality you all seek. As his vessel of abundance, I shall provide you with that nectar and many other things as well. Know that wherever there is wealth, good friends, plentiful crops and food, healthy children, and any other abundant circumstance, my blessing has made it so. Ever merciful, I hear the supplications of the worthy ones and respond with the swiftness of grace that every mother bestows upon her beloved children. Yet do not mistake my gentle nature for weakness. I have other manifestations that would make you tremble if you but knew of them. However, in this form as Lakshmi, my nature is to give to you abundantly."

"Yes," Indra rushed to interject his own authority in the midst of her words. "Whosoever pleases me, I will command her to give to that person in a most lavish way. I am, of course, quite generous by nature."

With the barest sparkle of amusement, the glowing figure of Lakshmi turned to him and spoke. "O most generous one, you are now going to demonstrate just how deep that vein of giving is rooted. For I am not to be your consort or your possession. You who are primarily concerned with your status and position must dedicate all your talent and energy to maintaining that place. I am meant for another, whose sole concern is for the welfare of the righteous ones. I speak, naturally, of the noble Vishnu."

So saying, she glided over to Vishnu and placed her arm about his neck in an affectionate manner. Without hesitation his arm slipped around her waist and they unabashedly looked into each other's eyes with deep love and affection. The crowd gasped in mixed delight and envy, as the two exchanged delicate and sweet words with each other that only they could hear.

Then Lakshmi turned back to the crowd and spoke again, instructing them all. "My form is composed of vibration, as is every other form in the cosmos. Because my form is the nature of abundance, whosoever shall call my name through various mystic methods shall be rewarded. Those who want wealth will inevitably obtain it through speaking my mystic name with sincerity and devotion. Those who desire regal children of beauty and charm shall have them through the grace of the mantra powers derived from me. Still others who want love and liberation shall have it by the grace contained in the mystic spiritual formulas composing the vibrations of my form. All manner of *siddhis* (divine abilities) may be attained. But know that all of this is possible by the grace of that Being whose dreamlike thoughts have made this universe possible: Narayana. Indeed, I am in Him and He in Me."

Lakshmi paused briefly to let her last remark sink in, then continued. "I now charge the compassionate Vishnu with every power available to complete his appointed divine task from now until the end of time and beyond." With that, she rapidly grew smaller until she was no bigger than one's closed hand. She melted into the chest of Vishnu, throbbing as part of his own celestial heart from which a blazing strand of light then slipped down his spine to its very base, paused briefly and moved up once again to his head, filling it with spidery tendrils of golden energy.

Vishnu stood wrapped in bliss, shedding tears of joy, and spoke without even hearing his own voice: "God's love, through whatever door it comes, is the end of all desire and yearning." And with that he walked away, steeped in the growing knowledge of his role and power in the new, material universe that was quickly emerging from the great churning that had come to an end. He had everything he needed to serve sentient beings for the next thousand, thousand millennia by the power of the Great Feminine. Lakshmi, residing in his heart, had linked to the great shakti lying in serene repose at the base of his spine. By so joining, she had supercharged Vishnu in every way. A tiny filament of light-borne shakti entered the Kaustubha Gem just below Vishnu's throat and it glowed magnificently.

Shiva smiled broadly at Parvati, who reached over and clenched his hand. "This is going to be fun," Shiva said softly to her. Parvati nodded and replied, "The power of her mystic name and mantras will propel millions of souls from this material universe to the divine shore."

Linked with Vishnu, Lakshmi would now incarnate with him whenever he descended to the physical plane to protect the pious ones and restore *dharma* (divine law). With Rama she would be Sita, with Krishna she would be Radha his ecstatic lover as well as Rukmini, his divine bride, as told in Chapter 8. With the Buddha she would be with him only in spirit, as Tara, and with Kulki she would also be Rukmini, as well as his thousand powers. Saraswati's words would be fulfilled, but wherever Vishnu manifests, there she would be, one way or another.

Indra, displeased at his abandonment, hissed at no one in particular, "What's the point of being chief of the celestials if I am treated this way."

"Careful," said Shiva. "You know full well that you can be replaced as chief. Be on guard! But do not worry, I will help you."

Vishnu, turning back briefly, also spoke to Indra. "As our noble leader, you constantly fight the demons. It is a thankless task. Therefore, I will always be available to come to your assistance in times of difficulty. Further, I will always honor you in your status as chief of all the celestials. No matter what happens, I will not desert you."

Indra bowed his head. "I hear your supportive words, Vishnu, and have no doubt that the benevolent and generous power of Lakshmi has inspired you in this way. I therefore honor you as her choice as if it were my very own, and express heartfelt gladness at your expression of friendship and support. Further, wherever Lakshmi's praises are sung or spoken, I will shed rain and proper winds to help the crops grow properly. In whatever way I can further the benevolence of Lakshmi, I shall do so."

In the coming millennia, even though Indra retained his position and title as chief of the celestials, sadly his fame slipped from a position of prominence into one of relative obscurity. Today, it is Vishnu, Shiva, and Brahma who are well known, while only scholars and priests remember and honor Indra. But when celestial battles are fought it is Indra who leads opposition to the negative forces of destruction, and Vishnu is beside him, true to his word. Wherever the praises of Lakshmi are chanted or sung, Indra lends ease to the situation through those means available to him, as he said he would. Indeed, the Maha Lakshmi Astakam hymn chanted even today is said to have been composed by Indra.

Emerging then from the raptured daze Lakshmi had produced in them, the celestials and the demons began to realize that the Nectar of Immortality still had not appeared. Suddenly, from out of the whirling blaze there appeared an unknown sage walking across the newborn stars carrying an urn. He smiled a radiant beam of invigorating energy, and all felt uplifted at the sight of him. As he neared the assembly, he spoke.

"It is true that I am unknown to you, but that which I carry is what you seek. I am Dhanvantari who has been created through the grace of Lakshmi. My job is that of physician and healer. In this jug is the Nectar of Immortality that has caused you all to perform such a great task as churning this ocean of consciousness and bringing the physical universe into being. Please now line up—mind you no fighting, pushing, or shoving—and I will give you each a draft."

Obediently, the gathering of celestials and demons formed a line and in due course each received a portion of the precious liquid.* To keep them from becoming impatient as they waited their turn, Dhanvantari spoke to them of plants and herbs that would be useful to all in the new universe. He also chanted mantras and recited various fire and water disciplines that would relieve a variety of conditions. He concluded his discourse when the last demon and celestial had received a cupful of the Nectar of Immortality.

"Lakshmi is the one who has brought me here. It is through her grace that healing methods and the recovered nectar have been brought forth by your efforts. As an emanation of her abundance, I entreat you to ever sing her praises and never forget the bounty she has given to all today. Fortunate are we that she has promised that from this day forward she will deliver a full measure of her abundance to all who genuinely seek it."

Nodding their agreement, both demons and celestials turned away and scattered into the cosmos. Some retained their etheric existence while others dove into the ocean of the emerging material universe to experience this thing called physicality. But none would forget the radiant abundance of Lakshmi and her promise to all sentient life.

---

*In another version of this story the demons stole the nectar and Vishnu retrieved it from them.

Lakshmi's Bounty for Us

The story of Lakshmi's appearance conveys the essence of the journey of spiritual growth we all take sooner or later. In you and me, the churn of the ocean of consciousness is the conscious, self-willed transformational process in which we engage to produce spiritual growth. The Vedas and other Eastern spiritual texts all conclude that the end result of any truly spiritual transformational process is immortality. When we plow deep down into the recesses of our own mind during whatever form of meditation in which we are engaged, sooner or later we will probably encounter foul things, just as poison from the serpent Vasuki was the first result of the churning in the story.

In Western literature, the transformational journey of Dante the Pilgrim in *The Divine Comedy* is an allegory with a similar outcome. Much more than the social and political allegory it is sometimes portrayed to be, *The Divine Comedy* shows Dante as "everyman" plowing deep into the recesses of his own subconscious mind, the "Inferno." Dante the Pilgrim's only protection is Virgil, the power of a rational mind guided by faith. Finally, just as Lakshmi appears from the churning of the ocean of consciousness to empower Vishnu, Beatrice appears to Dante and inspires him while explaining that God sent her to guide and bless him.

In my own meditations I have encountered many things within that reminded me of Dante's journey through Hell or Vasuki's poison. For if any of us plunge deep into our subconscious with single-minded spiritual purpose, unpleasant deeds we have performed in other lives, long held captive in subconscious memory, may be liberated and bubble up to be encountered by our conscious mind. We must face these things, forgive them, and go on. It is only by forgiving ourselves that we have the strength of

compassion to forgive others in a powerful, deep, and meaningful way.

The Nectar of Immortality, sought by celestials and demons
alike, also exists within us at the *Soma* chakra, situated just above
the brow center between the eyes. In this esoteric chakra, an etheric nectar collects. When stimulated, it flows, dripping into the
nadis or subtle channels that permeate our etheric form, permanently clearing away all karma, making that body immortal. Himalayan yogis know about this hidden nectar within and ardently
strive to maximize the flow of this magical liquid, knowing that
wherever it flows karma is permanently eradicated. Indeed, those
lonely ascetics practice a whole set of strange physical disciplines
designed to stimulate the flow of this liquid from its resting pool
in the Soma chakra.

Perhaps you may have experienced the flow of this precious
and subtle liquid as it splashes in small, dripping movements in your
subtle body. It feels as if slightly cool water may have moved two or
three inches down your leg or arm. But when you look, there is no
wetness at all, because it has dripped *inside* your body, not outside.

Lakshmi also exists within us at the heart or Anahata chakra,
holding ten qualities that she can release in us through her connection with the activity of the powerful shakti sitting at the base
of the spine. Those ten qualities are food, royal power, mystic
power of manifestation, universal sovereignty, noble rank, holy
luster, kingdom, fortune, bounteousness, and beauty.

Because the heart chakra, as the abode of Lakshmi, is said to ra-
diate beauty, Lakshmi has come to be associated with the beauty
of a lotus flower. The symbology of the lotus flower is important
in another way as well. Springing from the fetid recesses of a stag-
nant pond, the lotus is often used as an example of how something sublimely beautiful can emerge from something ugly and
distasteful. In us, the flower of great spiritual progress can emerge

from the mud and muck of our karma, if we will but make consistent efforts to improve and grow. For century upon centuries, Indian sages have taught that even our most foul karma can make blossom the shining bounty of Lakshmi.

Padma, another name associated with Lakshmi, means "flower" and is often given to girl children in Hindu families to denote that she carries the bounty of Lakshmi within her. Padma also means "chakra." Padma/Lakshmi carries an energy that can activate every positive attribute held in potential in all of our chakras.

Lakshmi Lady

Doe Lang, who lives in New York City, is the closest to a living example of Lakshmi that my wife, Margalo, and I have ever seen. The idea and manifestation of abundance oozes from her. For many years she has been teaching, lecturing, and advising clients and students, helping them reach their own joyful and abundant self within. Her book, *The Secrets of Charisma,* has sold over 100,000 copies, but that does not really convey what she does for her students and friends. Everyone whose life she touches becomes transformed in some way. For some it is simple self-acceptance. For others, their careers blossom as they start to believe in themselves. Still others just find that good things start to happen to them.

One example of how the universe responds to Doe stands out vividly in memory even though it occurred nearly twenty years ago. A small group of us were gathered to play a brand-new, guided, New Age self-discovery board game. When the half-dozen players had gathered, the game facilitator told us how to select our personal game pieces. She also explained we would be playing from four to six hours to get the true effects and proper feedback from the universe that would come through the game. At her second turn, after we had been playing for about twenty minutes, Doe's turn took her on a journey through several dizzying phases of the game activity. With each passing turn of events, the facilitator looked more and more perplexed. Finally, Doe arrived at a place where the game declared, through one of its special cards, that Doe was the epitome of all that was abundant and good, and that the highest good fortune would always accompany her. With that, the game declared that she was finished.

With an enthusiastic but very puzzled demeanor, the facilitator revealed that very few people *ever* attained this place, and those who reached it arrived only after playing the game several times, for several hours each time. The fact that Doe had reached this place in twenty minutes was something for which the facilitator was completely unprepared. With a mystified look on her face, she said that there was nothing more the game could give or show Doe. Knowing her, I think her name should be Doe "Lakshmi" Lang.

The Available Abundance of Lakshmi

Narayana sent Lakshmi to our physical universe to be the bestower of every form of abundance. We can also invoke that never-ending harvest of good qualities. We can bring all that is abundant, good, and noble and pure into our own lives by the grace of the Great Feminine.

In the story, Lakshmi proclaims herself available through the mystic formulas that vibrate with her essence. There are mantras that invoke Lakshmi to remedy any lack of material abundance, as well as to help us become an extension of her heart-centered, great aspect: Maha Lakshmi. With these mantra formulas there is no lack we cannot answer abundantly.

Although within the great spiritual teachings of the East there are thousands of names and mantras that pertain to Lakshmi, a handful of names for this feminine principle contain the most important of her powers that we may wish to invoke in ourselves.

To Ensure Enough Food to Eat

Having enough food to eat is a basic necessity to human existence. The Buddha and Mahatma Gandhi both knew that a hungry person cannot be taught how to meditate. The basic need for nourishment must be satisfied first. This mantra will set forces into motion to ensure you have enough food. If you decide to use this mantra in service to others, chanting for instance to end world hunger, begin your individual or group mantra work with an opening prayer like: "Without taking on the karma of any hungry being, I ask that through this mantra work, hunger in this world be abated for all beings who suffer this deprivation."

1. Om Shrim Lakshmiyei Swaha
[Om Shreem Lahk-shmee-yea Swah-ha]
"Om and salutations to She who provides abundance."

To Invoke Financial Prosperity

All of us have encountered circumstances where more money could have alleviated problems. Maybe it was some unexpected illness that created huge medical bills that could not be paid right away. Perhaps a family member experienced a sudden job reversal or other predicament that would have been easily solved by an infusion of cash. Sometimes there are friends or family members who are struggling to begin a new career. A loan or gift could help them over a rough spot or even make the whole enterprise doable and not just a dream. These kinds of situations appear all the time. Now you have powerful spiritual tools, in the form of these mantras, to help in situations like these that suddenly require more money.

To produce abundance, the mantra below should be practiced intensely for a minimum of forty days. During that time, you may find your mind directed to embark upon some new activities or to abandon others that you had planned on doing. Allow your intuition to guide you. Consider that you are actually changing your karma by your efforts, so things will be changing in your life. Be open and willing to discard some activities and welcome new ones. This powerful mantra has already helped many (including me) to attain new levels of prosperity.

Please remember that benefits of endowment with other of the ten regal qualities (food, royal power, mystic power, universal sovereignty, noble rank, holy luster, kingdom, fortune, bounteousness, and beauty) may also accrue from your practice of this mantra. So if new authority comes your way through work or in a service organization, be grateful and pray to use your new authority wisely.

2. Om Shrim Maha Lakshmiyei Swaha
[Om Shreem Mah-hah Lahk-shmee-yea Swah-hah]
"Om and salutations to She who provides abundance."

A reader of my first book, *Healing Mantras,* in which this mantra also appears, wrote the following: "I looked for months for a new job with no success. On December 23 [1999] I began reading this book and [began chanting]. . . . On January 23 I received a call from someone I barely knew but had worked with seven years ago. He had heard I was looking for a new job and asked me to meet him that day to discuss one he had available. It was even better than what I had been looking for—interesting work in a field I enjoy, better salary, better benefits, opportunity for advancement, and a great location. I received an offer on January 31, exactly 40 days after I began the mantra."

To Become More Attractive

Although we all know that physical beauty manifests in surface features, it is also well known that true beauty lies within. Therefore, no matter what our outward appearance, we can generate such beauty from within that ultimately our outward appearance matters less and less. We may actually seem to become more physically handsome or attractive. After a substantial period of time devoted to chanting of the right mantras, all people will see when they look at us is our inner beauty. It is this inner beauty that the following mantra increases.

3. Om Padma Sundharyei Namaha
[Om Pahd-mah Soon-dhar-yea Nahm-ah-hah]
"Om and salutations to She who personifies beauty."

To Make the Personality More Pleasing

When Lakshmi melted into his heart, Vishnu's nature changed. Even though he was noble in thought and action to begin with, the depth of his change in those qualities was incalculable. Her grace and subsequent union with his heart enabled Lakshmi to become Vishnu's spouse, or *patni* in Sanskrit. Thereafter, his already noble personality changed and became gentle and pure in every way without relinquishing power. The following mantra will similarly bestow pleasing qualities upon your personality. Although it is a long mantra, you will find that it is easy to learn and a delight to say. Early in my career as a spiritual teacher, I used this mantra to help erase any blemish on my personality that might stand in the way of my doing my job properly.

4. Om Maha Lakshmicha Vidmahae
Vishnu Patnicha Dhimahi

Tanno Lakshmi Prachodayat
[Om Mah-hah Laksh-mee-chah Veed-mah-hae
Vish-noo Paht-nee-chah Dee-mah-hee
Tah-no Laksh-mee Prah-cho-dhah-yaht]
"Om and salutations to that primordial Lakshmi, spouse
of Vishnu, kindly impel us toward that elevated state you
represent."

To Develop the Powers of Lakshmi

The ten qualities of Lakshmi are a mine of personal treasure
as well as a boon to society in general. Thus, if you are a person
who works in business or government, this mantra will help you
smooth out problems in situations in which you are involved.
Chant this mantra to bring the power of wisdom and other of
Lakshmi's attributes to your surroundings. Your leadership, founded
on compassion and steeped in right thinking, may be just the in-
gredient to positively affect hundreds or even thousands of lives.

5. Om Shrim Siddhayei Namaha
[Om Shreem Sid-hah-yea Nahm-ah-hah]
"Om and salutations to She who releases magical abilities
within."

To Invoke and Produce the Peace of Lakshmi

There are times when peace, in its dynamically powerful application, is the only remedy that will satisfy a current problem. But
someone must be the vessel of that peace. There must be a person
who has developed the capacity to carry that great peace that automatically calms any situation and which by its very nature begins to restore reason. If you desire to become such a person, then
this mantra will be invaluable to you in your service to others.

6. Om Shantiyei Namaha
[Om Shahn-tee-yea Nahm-ah-hah]
"Om and Salutations to She who is the giver of peace."

To Produce in Oneself the Spirit of Truth

In addition to peace, the spirit of truth is a powerful antidote for many difficult situations. Where deceit and false statements manipulate people and events, the spirit of truth can reveal the intentions and practices of those who distort for their own purpose. While tumult may temporarily result from these revelations, such exposure must take place if fair dealings, good government, and honest treatment of workers is to be restored. There are some of you who are destined to be part of the noble and good forces operating in business and government, as well as other mechanisms that operate in society. For people involved in occupations in corporations or government, an invincible spirit of truth is an invaluable ally. That spirit of truth can act as a shield against intrigue and a buffer against deception designed to undermine your position. To become a vessel for the spirit of truth helpful to all, dedicate yourself to this mantra.

7. Om Satyei Namaha
[Om Saht-yea Nahm-ah-hah]
"Om and salutations to She who empowers truth."

To Attune with the Celestial Healer

In the story, Dhanvantari, the celestial healer, appeared carrying a jug of the Nectar of Immortality and attributed his existence to the grace of Lakshmi. Today the mantra of Dhanvantari is practiced for two objectives. If you would like to embark upon a healing profession or increase your effectiveness as a healer, this mantra is for you. Second, if you have some affliction or condition and are unsure of the proper course of treatment, this mantra can help guide you to a remedy or treatment path appropriate to the problem. In India, women often chant this mantra over food prepared for family members who are ill or infirm.

I once taught this mantra to a class as just one of many, many mantras covered during the course. During a guided meditation, one of the class members had an unexpected vision of this mythic figure and experienced an epiphany regarding a physical problem she had been struggling with for years.

8. Om Shri Dhanvantre Namaha
[Om Shree Dhahn-vahn-trea Nah-ma-hah]
"Om and salutations to the celestial healer."

To Invoke and Eventually Become the Abundance of the Universe Itself

There are those among us who are so completely giving by nature that to be around them is to become joyful, just as the appearance of Lakshmi wiped all cares from the minds of those who first beheld her. We all need such people in our lives today, and perhaps you are one of them. Vishnu spoke these words in the story: "God's love, through whatever door it comes, is the end of all desire and yearning." The highest abundance is Love. If you feel that your true inner nature is one with the loving abundant nature of Lakshmi, that you want to bring an abundantly satisfied state of mind to every person and thing you encounter, these two mantras can begin the process of your transformation into such a bountiful and beneficent state. Although there is a separate mantra for Divine Love found at the end of this book, these Lakshmi mantras powerfully develop the power of the heart's love.

9. **Om Shrim Maha Lakshmiyei Swaha (age twenty-nine and older)**
[Om Shreem Mah-hah Lahk-shmee-yea Swah-hah]

Om Shrim Maha Lakshmiyei Namaha (age twenty-nine and younger)
[Om Shreem Mah-hah Lahk-shmee-yea Nah-mah-hah]
"Salutations to She who is that Great Abundance we salute and invoke."

Anasuya—Perfect Vessel of Lakshmi

Among the ten great sages, who are collectively called the Prajapati, is Atri whose wife, Anasuya, shares his exalted state of consciousness. After years of study and meditation, the highest mysteries of Lakshmi were revealed to Anasuya and she became contented beyond any human measure. A story about Anasuya describes how the Hindu Masculine Trinity—Brahma, Vishnu, and Shiva—came to test and confirm her spiritual attainment. Knocking upon her door, they appeared disguised as three travelers and begged for food. Knowing the ancient tradition that God may come as an unknown and unannounced guest, Anasuya invited the three men in.

As she started to leave the room to prepare food for them, one of the trio insulted her in the worst way possible, asking her to serve them while she was naked. Unperturbed for even a moment, Anasuya inquired if that was indeed what they desired. They agreed that this was exactly what they desired. She should serve them food while undressed.

Going to a nearby jug of water that she had used to perform a *puja* (religious ceremony) to Lakshmi earlier that day, she returned with a few drops of water in the palm of her hand. Before they could analyze what she was doing, she sprinkled a few drops of water over them. Instantly, they were reduced to infants, whereupon she opened her sari and fed each from her breast.

In the *Lakshmi Tantra*, the goddess of abundance teaches any who will listen, "In this universe of forms, there is only me. When I look out through your eyes and see another person, it is really me looking at myself. Through your eyes, I behold the glories of this universe that is my own abundance in diverse forms. Therefore, identify yourself with me and become everything."

5

Durga and Chamundi
The Power of Protection

Whether we are aware of it or not, every path of every human being is a spiritual path, and every path is both personal and individual. Although surely the spiritual aspect of some paths are
extremely well disguised, sometimes almost in spite of ourselves
we are all growing spiritually. When our lessons have finally been
learned, we will become a divine species. But as we presently grope
our way along, by day or by night, we occasionally find ourselves
in a situation where we feel nervous, fearful, or even panicky.

Have you ever been in a parking lot in an unsavory part of
town at night and you are just the slightest bit nervous? I have.

Have you ever been in your own home and seen something
just out of the corner of your eye that made you feel uneasy, but
when you turned toward it there was nothing there? I have.

Have you ever had dreams that caused you agitation, even
upon waking, because of someone or something you encountered
in the dream? I have.

And these dim, often insubstantial threats are not the only sort
we encounter. We may at some point in our lives become entan-
gled with a person who has severely unpredictable mood swings

or violent tendencies. We may encounter someone at work who is jealous of our career progress or of our seemingly better relationship to the powers that be.

It is in circumstances like these that I use mantras to invoke the protective powers of the great feminine forces of Durga or Chamundi. Durga can channel a potent mix of all-animating Para Shakti, Kriya Shakti (the power of mind over matter), and Iccha Shakti (the power of will). She will protect us from external harm with the ferocity of a lioness guarding her cubs.

Used over time, the mantras associated with the Goddesses Durga and Chamundi produce two profound results. The first is a kind of vibrational protective armor that shrugs off attempts to enter our lives and world through intrigue or actual opposition to us. The other result is much more subtle. It is as if a field of proactive intelligence guards us from negative persons or circumstances.

The Birth of Durga—Chamundi

You will recall from the story of Saraswati that two demons threatened Brahma just as he was being born. Rather than destroy them, Lakshmi banished the two to a far point in the universe. Of course she knows, as do we, that the evil will return one day.

Many thousands of cycles later, one of those two demons, now incarnated as Mahi Asura, performed a great spiritual discipline that resulted in gains of unconquerable strength. Armed with terrible might, he engaged some of the celestials in battle to test his prowess and was easily victorious. It seemed to Mahi Asura that he now had a chance to establish a foothold in all parts of the celestial spheres. So he led the rest of the demons in war upon the celestial forces and defeated an army led by Indra. Again, Saraswati's words came to pass.

One by one Mahi Asura took control over jobs previously performed by the celestials, gaining rulership of the moon and control of the eight cardinal directions. Forced to flee, the celestials were finally forced to the Earth plane, where they disguised themselves as ascetics and hermits and disappeared into the throngs of humanity. Secretly, so as not to be discovered by the demon forces, a delegation of thirty celestials took their case first to Vishnu.

Indra spoke first. "O, compassionate one who is revered by all, we need your help." Indra held great respect for Vishnu, who had made good his pledge on more than one occasion to aid him in his job as chief of the celestials.

Another celestial, Varuna, continued, "This Mahi Asura has gained great power from someplace. He is not just another tiresome fellow with wicked ways and insatiable appetites. He apparently has something more. "

"Hmmmmmm," pondered Vishnu. "Has anyone here more information?" he asked. At first the celestials remained silent. Then Lakshmi spoke. "Many cycles ago, when the universe was so young that expansion had not yet begun, I encountered one who bears a striking resemblance to this Mahi Asura."

"Can you tell us anything about the extent of his power?" asked Vishnu.

"I cannot," replied Lakshmi. "When I first met him he was just an ordinary troublemaker who entreated me to let him live. I could not refuse. In a sense, I fear I am somewhat responsible for the present state of affairs."

"Not at all, most regal one." Indra was still exceedingly fond of Lakshmi even though she had chosen Vishnu over him. "Your most compassionate nature would not allow you to do otherwise. Besides, how could you know that somehow he would gain such power?"

Lakshmi smiled and said to Vishnu so that only he could hear, "If they only knew that this was then foreseen." Turning to Indra,

Lakshmi spoke more loudly. "Your faith in me is both noble and touching. I can say this much with the authority Narayana has given me. This crisis shall be weathered and you shall prevail. It is up to you to determine how it will be accomplished."

"Since he is always impartial in such matters, I suggest we go to Lord Shiva," said Vishnu. "As the quintessential consciousness of everything, he will certainly be able to correctly advise us."

The celestials all quickly agreed and without further delay they mounted their respective vehicles and made off toward Mount Kailas, in the Himalayas, where Shiva and Parvati dwelled. Arriving in just a few minutes, they were astonished to see Parvati already laying out an ample spread of tea and sweets. "News travels fast in this cosmos," she joked, vanishing inside the cottage just as Shiva emerged to join them.

"So good to see you, although I wish the circumstances were more pleasant," Shiva said. "Tell me, how can I help?" He reached up and stroked the sleepy snake that lay coiled around his neck.

Vishnu spoke for the assembly. "We know that Mahi Asura has accumulated a significant store of spiritual power. But we are unsure of where he got it or how. Thus, we are at a loss concerning how best to relieve him of it or neutralize it. We beg your counsel."

Going inward for a second, Shiva spoke. "It was a boon, received from a very powerful source due to a monumental spiritual discipline he completed. His power was a reward."

Vishnu narrowed his eyes. "But who could have given such a boon? I tell you clearly it was not me. Lakshmi, was it you?"

"Not at all. Once is enough," replied Lakshmi.

"Lord Shiva, it is well known that you are impartial in matters of consciousness, was it you, perchance?" Vishnu inquired with respect.

"No, in truth, it was not me. Neither has Parvati dispensed such a powerful boon to anyone. I suspect that it is Brahma you seek. Here, let us ask him." Shiva lifted his chin and with deep resonance chanted, "Om Sat Chid Ekam Brahma."

Immediately Brahma appeared before them. "Who is it who calls so beautifully?" inquired the grandfather of sages.

"It was I, Grandfather," replied Shiva. "Please sit, have some tea. We have a question I think only you can answer."

Brahma was pleased at the invitation and noted the august gathering as he stirred sugar into his tea. "My, my, quite a select group we have here. What is the occasion?"

Vishnu was about to speak when Indra interrupted him. "Lord Brahma, did you give Mahi Asura a boon that granted him great power? He has beaten us all in battles that he, himself, started and we are reduced to hiding from him lest we experience yet another defeat at his hands. Come tell us, did you aid him?"

Brahma appeared crestfallen. "You did not invite me here to honor me, I can see that. You have some quarrel?" He looked around the group of celestials who sat mute at his question. He teetered on the brink of righteous disgust.

"No one ever has a quarrel with you, Grandfather," assured Shiva. "It is just that not having your infinite knowledge of the cosmos, there are times when we have questions that only you can answer. We only beg your advice. Nothing more."

Brahma calmed down and poured some cream into his tea, looking at it swirl into the brown mixture. "Looks just like the creation of the universe if you stir slowly enough," he commented, apparently absorbed in the contents of his cup.

No one else said so much as a single word. They just waited him out.

At length Brahma spoke once more. "Mahi Asura completed

one of the most strenuous spiritual disciplines I have ever seen. You all know that whosoever practices such disciplines and austerities shall gain great power through my favor. It is part of the very fabric of the laws that govern the cosmos. I evaluate various efforts and mete out rewards impartially, so do not blame me for this current state of affairs. I don't see any of you performing great spiritual disciplines. It could just as easily have been one of you. But it wasn't, was it?"

The silence was palpable as the celestials felt the truth of Brahma's words, and it stung.

"Nonetheless," sighed Brahma compassionately, "I will give you some assistance. The boon I gave Mahi Asura was that no one but a woman could defeat him. Mahi Asura thought this laughable and was satisfied in every way."

As this revelation sunk in, each of the celestials could not help but wonder aloud why none of them had completed a great discipline. In hindsight, it seemed that Indra, at least, should have done some kind of discipline. Catching the drift of their thought, Indra agreed, "It is my responsibility. I should have completed a great discipline just as Grandfather has said. I apologize to you all. Even though I am constantly engaged in activities for your welfare, I have no excuse. I should have done something." Indra was not at all pleased with himself and his face showed it.

"I, for one, have no complaint, Indra," said Shiva. "I have never seen you take a day of rest, nor cease in your efforts to lead us and work for our welfare in every way. No, I shall not accept your self-blame."

As the center of attention began to circulate among the celestials looking for a new scapegoat, Shiva spoke again. "Why do you not leave off this bickering and seek to combine your forces in some practical way?"

Vishnu, ever in communion with Lakshmi, noted that it is the feminine nature of things that provides all power, everywhere in the cosmos. Perhaps that might provide a key. "It is She who weaves the fabric of this creation at every level," said Vishnu. "Thus it is to Her we must make our supplication."

"A fire ceremony," said Indra immediately. "We need to perform the most powerful fire ceremony ever seen in this universe. Lord Shiva, may we use the neighboring valley to perform such a *yajna*?" (Yajna means, literally, sacrifice, but a sacrifice only of part of the ego in the name of something higher.)

"Of course," replied Shiva.

"I, too, wholeheartedly endorse such a ceremony," said Parvati. "In fact, I shall prepare certain herbs myself for you to throw into the fire."

There was a murmur at this. To have Parvati participate in such a way was an enormous blessing!

So it was that thirty of the most powerful and influential celestials created a huge fire ceremony to regain their rightful places in the cosmos. They drew upon all the principles connected with both energy and sound, as well as with deep understanding of the nature of sacred rituals to all the powers.

- They engaged in *Vishatkare*—the principle of sacrificial observances.
- They employed *Swara*—the ruling principle of sound, both obvious and subtle.
- They invoked *Swadha*—the ruling principle of the power of mantras.
- They practiced *Swaha*—the invocation and supplication power for mantras.

For many days and nights the fire raged, with each of the celestials adding something of their own essence to the fire. From the mouths of each of the thirty celestials a great burst of energy shot out, which mingled and combined dramatically, until, from this combining energy, a feminine form took shape over the leaping flames. Immediately, the form became conscious and discovered her own power.

The power of Shiva was in her face, the power of Vishnu moved into her many arms, the power of Brahma surged into her feet, and all other celestials were represented as power in her other parts. She was at once wondrous, beautiful, and terrible to behold. In the *Markandeya Purana* it is said that the full investiture of powers in her would take hundreds of pages just to describe in the briefest of terms.

Now that her magnificent power had been awakened and taken form, the sages, rishis, and munis offered prayers of supplication, asking for her protection from the demons that had taken over the etheric realm.

Smiling beatifically and brandishing weapons of destruction in her numerous hands, she presented a picture of powerful contrasts. When she smiled, a luminous and seductive radiance emanated from her, yet her countenance also held the unmistakable glint of a voracious appetite for battle.

Still, the celestials continued their thundering mantras, and Parvati's potent herbs were thrown into the raging fire. At this, a tiger appeared under the figure shaking its massive head back and forth. The tiger easily held her on its back, without being the least hampered in its ability to swipe a huge paw at prey or take a large bite from an enemy.

Indra spoke for all assembled, saying, "Make us victorious, O Devi, O Divine Feminine One, source of all power, Durga, who, in your capacity to delude, is difficult to see when ready to do battle."

Looking around at the gathered celestials, she spoke for the first time. "Although I was created by your powers, combining from your joined efforts, know that I am wholly independent. I will belong to no one. I am the spouse of none of you. To think that I am an instrument of your bidding would be the gravest mistake."

"O Durga, Chamundi, most powerful of all, we honor your presence among us and offer ourselves as your devotees," improvised Indra, with devotion and a very quick mind. "Knowing that you go wherever you please and do as you will, be merciful to us in our predicament. Since you have emerged from each of us in some way, you know the terrible situation that exists. Pray aid us in defeat of the demons that have wrongfully assumed power in the etheric realms."

Nodding curtly at those present, she whom they called Durga or Chamundi took off into the sky in search of the demons. No further explanation was necessary. What the celestials knew, she also knew.

Just as the demons were bedding down for the night, they spied a blaze of light in the sky. Suspecting some form of counterattack from the celestials, the demons quickly assembled for battle. As Durga astride her tiger rode closer, the demons recognized the various powers of the celestials of whom she was composed. They had triumphed over these powers before and assumed they would again be victorious. They were, of course, quite mistaken.

I will spare you the details of war, since they are the same in any war at any time. Carnage is always carnage. Durga's victory was accomplished with an ease rarely seen in mortal conflict. She returned then to the celestials who praised her mightily with the hymn that follows.

The variety of attributes this hymn consigns to Durga-Chamundi conveys what the celestials understood about the extent of her power.

Not only for battle, but for every force animating consciousness, she is praised as the Great Feminine. Because this most famous hymn to Shakti has come down to us intact, we can begin
to get a small glimmer of the extent to which the Great Feminine
was revered by the ancient seers. Even today, all over India, this
hymn is chanted to invoke the power of the Great Feminine in
matters great and small.

The Devi Mahatmyam

1. **Namo Devyei Maha Devyei Shivayei Satatam Namaha
Prakrityei Bhadrayei Niyata Pranata Smatam**
"Salutations to the Great Feminine, who is the abode of all
blessings. Salutations to She who is the primordial energy
of the cosmos and its sustaining principle. We offer adorations with deepest devotion."

2. **Raudrayei Namo Nityayei Gauryei Dhatrayei Namo
Namaha Jyotsnayei Chandu Rupinyei Sukhayei Satatam
Namaha**
"Adorations to She who is both dreadful and eternal. She
is the bright one who sustains the cosmos with a soothing
form of the moon with its coolness, grace, and charm.
Salutations to the source of bliss again and again."

3. **Kalyanyei Pranata Vridyei Siddyei Kurmo Namo
Namaha Nairatyei Bhubritam Lakshmiyei Sharvanyei Te
Namo Namaha**
"Adorations to She who is the source of all blessings. She is
prosperity, success, and all forms of wealth. She is also the
misfortune of the arrogant ones as well as the Goddess of

Fortune to her votaries. The very consort of consciousness, we salute her again and again."

4. Durgayei Durga Parayei Sarayei Sarva Karineyi Khyatyei Tathaiva Krishnayei Dhumrayei Satatam Namo Namaha
"I make my deepest bows and offer my inner obeisance to the Great Feminine who takes her flock across the ocean of tribulations. She is the originator of all and the essence of everything. To She who often appears in a deep spiritual blue, I offer songs of praise."

5. Ati Saumya Atiraudrayei Nata Statsyei Namo Namaha Namo Jagat Pratistayei Devyei Krityei Namo Namaha
"Salutations to She who can be terrible when need be, but who is gentle by nature and upholds the Universe. She is the fountain of all creativity. To her we bow again and again."

6. Ya Devi Sarva Bhuteshu Vishnu Mayeti Shabdita Nama Stasyei Nama Stasyei Nama Stasyei Namo Namaha
"Salutations to the Great Feminine, power of Vishnu him-self, who abides in all beings. Salutations again and again. Here are but a few of your ineffable qualities."

7. Ya Devi Sarva Bhuteshu Cheteneya [Infinite Consciousness] Rupena Bhiditate Nama Stasyei Nama Stasyei Nama Stasyei Namo Namaha
"I bow to the Great Feminine who abides in all beings in the form of Infinite Consciousness."

8. Ya Devi Sarva Bhuteshu Buddhi [Intelligence] Rupena Samsthita Nama Stasyei Nama Stasyei Nama Stasyei Namo Namaha
"I bow to the Great Feminine who abides in all beings in the form of Intelligence."

9. Ya Devi Sarva Bhuteshu Nidra [Sleep] Rupena Samsthita Nama Stasyei Nama Stasyei Nama Stasyei Namo Namaha
"I bow to the Great Feminine who abides in all beings in the form of Sleep."

10. Ya Devi Sarva Bhuteshu Kshudhi [Hunger] Rupena Samsthita Nama Stasyei Nama Stasyei Nama Stasyei Namo Namaha
"I bow to the Great Feminine who abides in all beings in the form of Hunger."

11. Ya Devi Sarva Bhuteshu Chaya [Reflection] Rupena Samsthita Nama Stasyei Nama Stasyei Nama Stasyei Namo Namaha
"I bow to the Great Feminine who abides in all beings in the form of Reflection."

12. Ya Devi Sarva Bhuteshu Shakti [Power] Rupena Samsthita Nama Stasyei Nama Stasyei Nama Stasyei Namo Namaha
"I bow to the Great Feminine who abides in all beings in the form of Power."

13. Ya Devi Sarva Bhuteshu Thrishna [Thirst] Rupena Samsthita Nama Stasyei Nama Stasyei Nama Stasyei Namo Namaha

"I bow to the Great Feminine who abides in all beings in the form of Thirst."

14. Ya Devi Sarva Bhuteshu Kshanti [Forgiveness] Rupena Samsthita Nama Stasyei Nama Stasyei Nama Stasyei Namo Namaha
"I bow to the Great Feminine who abides in all beings in the form of Forgiveness."

15. Ya Devi Sarva Bhuteshu Jati [Genius] Rupena Samsthita Nama Stasyei Nama Stasyei Nama Stasyei Namo Namaha
"I bow to the Great Feminine who abides in all beings in the form of Genius."

16. Ya Devi Sarva Bhuteshu Laja [Modesty] Rupena Samsthita Nama Stasyei Nama Stasyei Nama Stasyei Namo Namaha
"I bow to the Great Feminine who abides in all beings in the form of Modesty."

17. Ya Devi Sarva Bhuteshu Shanti [Peace] Rupena Samsthita Nama Stasyei Nama Stasyei Nama Stasyei Namo Namaha
"I bow to the Great Feminine who abides in all beings in the form of Peace."

18. Ya Devi Sarva Bhuteshu Shraddha [Faith] Rupena Samsthita Nama Stasyei Nama Stasyei Nama Stasyei Namo Namaha
"I bow to the Great Feminine who abides in all beings in the form of Faith."

19. Ya Devi Sarva Bhuteshu Kanti [Beauty] Rupena Samsthita Nama Stasyei Nama Stasyei Nama Stasyei Namo Namaha

"I bow to the Great Feminine who abides in all beings in the form of Beauty."

20. Ya Devi Sarva Bhuteshu Vritti [Activity] Rupena Samsthita Nama Stasyei Nama Stasyei Nama Stasyei Namo Namaha

"I bow to the Great Feminine who abides in all beings in the form of Activity."

21. Ya Devi Sarva Bhuteshu Smritti [Memory] Rupena Samsthita Nama Stasyei Nama Stasyei Nama Stasyei Namo Namaha

"I bow to the Great Feminine who abides in all beings in the form of Memory."

22. Ya Devi Sarva Bhuteshu Daya [Compassion] Rupena Samsthita Nama Stasyei Nama Stasyei Nama Stasyei Namo Namaha

"I bow to the Great Feminine who abides in all beings in the form of Compassion."

23. Ya Devi Sarva Bhuteshu Tusti [Contentment] Rupena Samsthita Nama Stasyei Nama Stasyei Nama Stasyei Namo Namaha

"I bow to the Great Feminine who abides in all beings in the form of Contentment."

24. Ya Devi Sarva Bhuteshu Matri [Mother] Rupena Samsthita Nama Stasyei Nama Stasyei Nama Stasyei Namo Namaha

"I bow to the Great Feminine who abides in all beings in the form of the Mother."

25. Ya Devi Sarva Bhuteshu Bhranti [Delusion] Rupena Samsthita Nama Stasyei Nama Stasyei Nama Stasyei Namo Namaha
"I bow to the Great Feminine who abides in all beings in the form of Delusion."

26. Indriyanam Adhistatri Bhutanamcha Akilei Shucha Bhuteshu Satatam Tasyei Vyapti Devyei Namo Namaha
"I bow again and again to the rules of all the elements and senses. Salutations to the Great Feminine."

27. Chiti Rupena Ya Krits Nametat Vyapya Stitha Jagat Nama Stasyei Nama Stasyei Nama Stasyei Namo Namaha
"The Great Feminine resides in all beings in the form of consciousness and pervades all parts of the Universe, adorations to Her again and again."

Pleased with their devotion, Durga hovered over the glowing coals of what had once been a great fire. Carefully, she who some called Chamundi looked from face to face and what she saw there pleased her. There was no guile or strategizing for her help. There were no hidden agendas lurking in the quiet recesses of their minds. Only gratitude and relief. Finally, she spoke. "In the future, whenever evil becomes so powerful that you are overcome, chant my mantras and hymns and I will come to vanquish those who oppose you." Then, she disappeared.

All for One and One for All

You will recall that I said at the beginning of this chapter that we are growing into a Divine Species. While this is true enough, it is also true that we have many lessons that first must be absorbed on the road to that destiny.

One of these lessons is Unity. Currently, humanity is separated by a thousand emotional and cultural barriers, likes and dislikes, fears and prejudices, and so forth. In this story, the celestials learned, if only at a collectively unconscious level, that regardless of our individual power or prowess, evil can be truly defeated only when we are united.

The story of Durga-Chamundi also teaches that the Great Feminine power does not "belong" to any one person. The united celestials were shown that this power, while part of them, was something unto itself. There is a lesson here for every spiritual teacher and seeker. There will come a time when power becomes invested in us. The Great Feminine will manifest and solve our problems. But this power does not belong to us; it is shared. We honor that power by recognizing its own intelligence as the vehicle of the divine.

The Conclusion

Now let us return to our story. . . .

Peace reigned for many cycles as Durga retired to an unmanifest state existing in a twilight consciousness of divine equipoise. Finally, two demons, Shumbha and Nishumbha, came as reincarnations of Mahi Asura and his brother, and once again began conquering the celestials and taking over their positions, just as they had done a millennium ago. However, this time the celestials knew what to do: The thirty great celestials gathered once more in a forest glen to sing the praises of Durga-Chamundi.

The songs and praises went on for hours. Eventually, the celestials ended their chanting and waited for something to happen. But Chamundi did not appear as she had said she would. This was puzzling. With increasing agitation, the celestials talked among themselves and wondered what they should do next to gain her attention. What, they wondered, would secure her favor? After more discussion, a delegation was formed to begin a search for Durga. With glum faces and a less than hopeful attitude, they went off into the forest in search of she who had saved them before.

No more than fifty paces into the forest, the celestials came upon a clearing and heard the lush sounds of a stream accompanied by singing. Following the singing to the far end of the clearing, they came upon Parvati, who was washing out a sari in the cool, clear water.

She, the sum total of all energy in the universe at all levels, saw the celestial party, and spoke. "What are you doing here in the forest?"

The celestials babbled almost in unison that they were looking for Durga. They explained that a new crop of powerful demons had come and oppressed them. "She told us that if we sang her praises, she would come," noted Indra ruefully. "But we sang and sang and she did not appear. Thinking that she might be in the forest, an unlikely thing, we freely admit, we are nonetheless searching for her."

With a wave of Parvati's hand, the realm of time and space occupied by the celestials became fluid and malleable. Out of the flesh of Parvati's body emerged Durga. In just moments the transformation was complete, and Durga-Chamundi spoke. "I shall

save you as promised. Now go, and I shall return when I am finished." Bolstered in spirit, the search party returned to tell the
others.

Durga retired to the woods, communing with the forest spirits
and the little creatures that made their homes among the trees,
bestowing her unending compassion on the world of nature. Before long, however, her reverie was broken by the demon Shumbha,
who had received a report of her whereabouts from his scout. As
we have noted, Durga was exceptionally beautiful. This was not
lost on Shumbha, but he was not capable of any true feelings of
love. Only lust.

"You must choose between my brother, Nishumbha, and me,"
the demon slathered. "To one of us you will be queen."

"I will marry only he who defeats me in battle." Chamundi
laughed.

Another epic battle ensued and, need it be said, the demons
were defeated, and peace reigned again.

Again the celestials sang her praises, and, yes, again Durga
promised to return to overcome any evil that cannot be dispatched
by other means.

Literal demons, hideous to gaze upon, are fairly rare in our
contemporary times. Yet unfortunately we may encounter humans
at the lower end of their spiritual development who can be petty
or destructive in thought, word, and deed. If in your life you feel
yourself in danger or in need of protection, you can call upon
Durga using her mantras.

Mantra for General Protection

This mantra is one of the most commonly used Sanskrit formulas for general protective purposes. In *Healing Mantras*, I tell the
story of Rick, who chanted this mantra while attending a rock
concert. His ability to assist a woman who became suddenly ill

and help her to travel to the safety of her home was powered by Durga-Chamundi. She has come to my aid as well.

Throughout the year, I perform ceremonies and give workshops in dozens of places. In my travels, in which my wife, Margalo, often accompanies me, I meet all kinds of people, most of whom are such a delight that I consider meeting them one of the blessings God has bestowed upon me. One time in the early 1980s, however, I encountered someone who was not quite so pleasant. As I stood outside the mountain setting during a workshop break, a man in his late thirties who seemed a bit unbalanced approached me in a threatening manner and accosted me with insults. I could sense that he was itching for a fight of some kind, and he both startled and frightened me.

As I stood there wondering how I should handle this fellow, Margalo appeared seemingly from nowhere. Now you should know that Durga is a favorite goddess of Margalo, and she has chanted Durga mantras and seed sounds for many thousands of repetitions. As she passed beside me and moved in front of me, I could see fire in her eyes. Her face became taut and filled with an energy that I sensed could explode at any moment. "You have some problem?" she hissed at this fellow. "You want to pick some kind of fight? You just might get more than you bargained for!" She waited for a moment, her arms straight and ready at her sides.

This was a side of my wife that I had not seen before. She looked as if she could sock him and send him into outer space, but all she was doing was looking at him and breathing in a steady but powerful rhythm: the breath of Durga's tiger, ready to spring into action. The man's mouth gaped ever so slightly. He was completely unprepared for this. He acknowledged stammeringly that perhaps he had been misunderstood, that he was not seeking any kind of confrontation. (Not true, believe me!) With a few mumbled phrases, he excused himself and walked away.

Margalo turned around, composing herself, but with the spark of Durga still clearly coursing in her blood. "Good thing he backed down. He would not have liked the outcome at all." Then she looked at me with exquisite tenderness and said, "When I see someone coming after you while you are trying to do good, I feel I just have to protect you." I nodded appreciatively. I had just seen Durga, and I believed.

1. Om Dum Durgayei Namaha
[Om Doom Door-gah-yea Nahm-ah-hah]
"Salutations to She who is beautiful to the seeker of truth and terrible in appearance to those who would injure devotees of truth."

Heavy-Duty Protection

This mantra, commonly used in particularly dreadful circumstances, can also bestow blessings of creativity and good fortune. In addition, I know of several women who have used this mantra to increase their self-confidence with remarkable success. For that reason I have started to recommend it for those suffering from eating disorders or other maladies that may stem from a deep-seated insecurity or feelings of lack of self-worth.

2. Om Eim Hrim Klim Chamundayei Vicche Namaha
[Om I'm Hreem Kleem Chah-moon-dah-yea Vee-chei Nah-mah-hah]
"Om and salutations to She who is radiant with power and wisdom."

The mantra can also be beneficial for others we may encounter, even while it protects us, as exemplified by the following incident. During the year of 2000 I undertook a spiritual discipline of this Chamundi mantra. I worked strenuously toward the completion of the 125,000 repetitions that compose the classical discipline for anchoring the power of the mantra firmly within. In the fall of that year, Margalo and I traveled to Toronto, Canada, to give a workshop for the Yoga Teachers Federation of Ontario.

After the workshop, we were hosted by a freelance television producer-director, Nadine Schwartz, for discussion of various projects. Still talking well into the second day, we eventually went to dinner. After our meal, we were walking the several blocks back to Nadine's apartment when out of the shadows appeared a disheveled young woman who was clearly disturbed. For whatever reason, the woman singled me out from the group and focused her venom upon me. She spat forth insult after vile insult. Getting no reaction, she suddenly and unexpectedly walked up to me and hit me right in the chest.

Although I was certainly surprised by all of this, I was seized by a dynamic force of great quietude. I was completely calm. Without thinking, my right hand came up and formed a *mudra* (divine gesture) of blessing and I heard myself saying "Be peaceful." As the words left my mouth, I could feel a force come out of my hand and enter her. She became wide-eyed and stopped for a second. This was the opportunity for our party to change course and cross to the other side of the street. As we moved away, the woman began her shouts again, but now there was an empty quality to her words. The force behind them was gone.

I attribute what came through me to the power of Chamundi, complete with compassion. This woman was not to be harmed in any way. Even though the experience was unpleasant for me and the attack unwarranted, I was not to be harmed by it and neither was she. The energy of Chamundi manifested in just the right way appropriate to the situation. All of us moved away into the night realizing that something amazing had just happened.

The Durga Mantra for Manifold Blessings

This mantra, called the Durga Gayatri, will eventually produce a sublimely elevated state of consciousness. The Gayatri referred to here applies to the rhythm or meter of the mantra, and not the Gayatri Mantra discussed in the chapter on Saraswati.

3. Om Katya-inicha Vidmahei Kanya Kumari-cha Dhimahi Tanno Durgihi Prachodayat
[Om Kaht-yah-ee-nee-cha Veed-mah-hei Kahn-yah Koo-mah-ree-cha Dhee-mah-hee Tah-noh Door-gee-hee Prah-choh-dah-yaht]

6

Kali
The Power of Destruction of Negative Ego

If you are impatient in your worldly or spiritual pursuits, Kali is for you. She is the fast track, often on a bumpy road, to problem solution and spiritual advancement. When called by mantras that carry her vibrations, Kali responds with a direct power that often leads right through some cherished part of our ego attachments. Her power tools are the Kundalini Shakti (the power of spiritual electricity); the Kriya Shakti, the power to creatively affect the universe; and Iccha Shakti, the power of will that personally compels our physical movements and actions, while in the universe it causes the galaxies to rush away from one another into cosmic night. Although she puts "effective" before "gentle," it should also be noted that even in the midst of the sometimes turbulent effects she produces, Kali is a repository of great compassion. The great Indian guru Paramahansa Ramakrishna viewed his beloved Kali as kindness and beneficence itself. But that is not the common conception of her.

Mention the Hindu goddess Kali to someone who has a nodding acquaintance with Eastern philosophy and you get an immediate reaction. "Oh, she's the one with the garland of skulls." Or, "Isn't she the one who drinks the blood of her enemies and the one for whom animal sacrifices are done? Are they still doing those?" Or, "I know, she's the one with bright red eyes who sticks her tongue way out." And, "She's the one with a face as dark and as deep as space itself."

"Yes, that's right," I would confirm each of those responses. That is Kali, and they still do animal sacrifices in her name in remote places in India. But more is the pity because they have lost track of who Kali is, what she stands for, and what her purpose is.

There is a long-standing play on words concerning Kali and "time," which in Sanskrit is *kala*. The saying in the Far East is, "Nothing is as ruthless as kala except Kali." Time is called the most ravenous creature of all. It inevitably devours all, taking our youth as an appetizer, our midlife as the main course, and our old age for dessert. Finished with us for one incarnation, it calls our number and sends us to another cycle of death and then rebirth. Not at all limited to our puny human lifetimes, it also dictates the erosion of the Earth and inexorably consumes it, as well as the sun and the stars.

But that which consumes even kala is Kali, for she is the infinite receiver of all. The inky black look of Kali is the inky blackness of the void. In the cosmos, Kali is she to whom all the energy of the universe returns, devoid of form, aspect, or object. Kali is the void of the cosmos that gives birth to the next *Maha Kalpa*, or great cycle of another universe.

In the *Maha Nirvana Tantra*, Shiva praises Kali in the following way: "At the dissolution of things, it is kala [time] that will devour all. But it is Kali that devours even time, the original form and devourer of all things. Resuming yourself after the great dissolution, you retain your own nature, dark and devoid of form. There, you remain ineffable and inconceivable. Source of all forms, you are the multiform power of *Maya* [illusion], the beginning of all, creatrix, protectress, and destructress." The *Kamada Tantra* also takes the idea of Kali to a more cosmic extension. There she is described as attributeless, neither male nor female, but the sublime imperishable one of being, consciousness, and bliss.

But if this last is an accurate description, then from where did this current gruesome image come? Who is this ferocious Kali?

In the earliest references to her, Kali does not have such a terrible reputation. If we go back far enough in time, we find only one reference to Kali as a "tongue of fire." She is one of eight tongues of fire, in fact, and part of the activity of Agni, the god or principle of Fire. Of the eight tongues, hers was the most destructive, and she came to be called "Kali the Terrible," but still this referred only to an aspect of fire.

Later, she began to be depicted as a woman with disheveled hair, gaunt and fanged, riding on the back of a ghost and frequenting cremation grounds. She is also described in some sources as wearing a garland of skulls, her elongated tongue sticking out of her mouth, sometimes dripping blood. She may be covered with snakes, and she laughs loudly, inspiring fear in all within hearing.

There may be a very good explanation for the "besmirching," if such it be, of Kali's reputation. The Brahmin priests achieved for themselves a level of infamy for selling indulgences of every sort for at least two thousand years before the Catholic Church thought of doing so. For the right price, these priests would perform rituals to make it hail on your neighbors' crops or make *their* cattle become *your* cattle. A fearsome figure, such as Kali was eventually purported to be, would come in handy for manipulating pious but ignorant souls to the priests' own benefit and reward. A priest might be paid to invoke Kali on behalf of those who felt they required vengeance for a wrong done them. Or a priest might also be paid to invoke Kali for one's protection. That she was female was also useful in a society that held women as second-class citizens. Her unsavory iconography reinforced certain grimy prejudices already in place. While I have yet to uncover proofs of this surmising, the existence of a corrupt priest caste is factual and Kali would, unless somehow subverted, be a natural enemy to this group.

The true Kali is revealed in a simple story in the *Bhagavata Purana*. Here the leader of a band of thieves holds Kali as his Patroness Saint. Thinking to please her and secure her blessing, the thief kidnaps a young Brahmin lad. The head of this boy would make the perfect offering to Kali, or so the thief imagines. But the thief was ignorant of Kali's inner purpose. Nor did he comprehend the youth's level of consciousness.

The young man was sinless, with a bright aura and untainted by any negative ego whatsoever. As a result, when he was brought before the image of Kali and his clothes set on fire, it was the image of Kali that burned, not the lad. Infuriated that the thieves would try to harm the innocent youth, Kali emerged from the statue and killed the leader of the thieves and his entire band of followers. Throughout, the young Brahmin boy remained unharmed.

This is the real essence of Kali. She is the destroyer of negative ego. The more negative the ego, the greater the destruction. Even those who view Kali as the voracious warrior who can conquer demons by the square mile will readily admit that if you set a child upon the field of battle she will immediately hear its cry, go to it, and take it to her breast. Her attitude instantly transforms into that of a Mother who thinks only of the welfare of her children. It is surprising that so much is written about her and even practiced that runs counter to this truth.

As noted earlier, Paramahansa Ramakrishna saw Kali full of both love and knowledge and the source of everything. As Georg Feuerstein reports in *Tantra: Path of Ecstasy,* "Kali's devotees . . . experience her as a loving, nurturing and protecting mother. With tear-filled eyes and a longing heart, they invoke her as Kali Ma, asking for health, wealth and happiness as well as liberation. Like a doting mother, she bestows all boons upon her human children. Sri Ramakrishna prayed to Kali for the fruit of all Yogas and, as he confirmed, 'She has shown me everything that is in the Vedas, the Vedanta, the Puranas and the Tantras.' Toward her devotees, Kali always presents her most benign aspect. Even her destructive side is modulated in a benevolent way, as a force that removes all outer and inner obstacles, especially spiritual blindness, and grants the highest realization beyond time and space."*

Kali as Protectress

In the previous chapter, I told the story of Durga, who emerged from the powers of thirty great celestials and slew the demon Mahi Asura. In other versions of this tale, just as Durga is getting ready to do battle, it is Kali who emerges from her forehead and engages the demons in war.

In yet another story, Durga is invoked to do battle with a demon called Raktabija and his armies. Durga came to war accompanied by her band of feminine warriors called the *Matrikas*, or the Mothers. When the battle commenced, the Matrikas destroyed the armies of Raktabija, while Durga concentrated on Raktabija himself. But whenever Durga struck the demon and spilled blood, just like the hydra in the Greek myth of Hercules, a new Raktabija emerged from each drop of spilled blood. Soon there were hundreds of Raktabijas and they were multiplying by the second. With a muttered supplication, Durga transformed herself into Kali, who immediately drank the blood of every Raktabija, letting not one drop escape her. Generation after generation has handed

*Georg Feuerstein, *Tantra: The Path of Ecstasy* (Boston and London: Shambhala, 1998), page 38.

down this mythic tale, and thus Kali's reputation as the drinker of blood was secured. Among the goddesses who comprise the Great Feminine, Kali is the last line of defense for the worst evils. Where lesser powers fail, Kali overcomes.

In still another tale, while Kali is devouring the legions of an enemy horde, there is fear on both sides of the conflict that she will not stop there, but will continue and eventually devour the world. To ward off such an eventuality, Shiva smears himself with holy cremation ash and goes to lie down before her in the battle-field. Kali continues through the field, destroying and trampling until she finds that she is standing with one foot upon Shiva. As soon as she notices this, she sticks out her tongue in the manner in which she's most often portrayed. Some pundits have suggested that this gesture with the tongue is to be regarded as an act of contrition or embarrassment. But I do not agree. I have had my own experiences with Kali, and I can tell you that I believe she is pleased at the sight of Shiva and her tongue is a playful invitation and a sign that the battle is over. Rather than an act of contrition, it is a succulent invitation of the most intimate sort.

In the *Adbhuta Ramayana*, Kali appears through Sita, wife of the avatar Rama, and protects Rama. After Rama has defeated the demon king, Ravana, he and Sita are returning to Ayodhya where they will be installed on the throne and rule the kingdom. But just as they are entering the forest, another demon jumps out of hiding with the intention of killing Rama. Startled, Rama momentarily freezes. Instantly, Sita transforms into Kali and consumes the demon on the spot. This shows that Sita, who is an incarnation of Lakshmi, also has the potential to become Kali when necessary. This story provides a wonderful example of the mutability of the Great Feminine, who can appear in any form at any time according to the need of the situation.

When Shiva and Kali are depicted together, such as on the battlefield, Kali is always shown standing over him, securely in the superior place. The symbolic meaning is that consciousness acknowledges and honors her as divine energy and even submits to her so that he may be empowered. At the same time, Shiva is always able to calm Kali, no matter how angry or terrible she has become. He is pure universal consciousness, devoid of any kind of negative ego.

Sometimes Shiva and Kali are shown dancing wildly in the moonlight. The interplay of infinite energy and infinite consciousness knows no boundaries, and their dance, disturbing though it may appear to some, illustrates the limitlessness of this infinite pairing. When Shiva and Kali dance, the world trembles, or so it seems. Yet it is important to note that in none of the stories concerning this duo is there lasting damage from their more frenetic activities.

The *Malati Madhava* records one of their more earthshaking dances near a local Kali temple. The dance is so violent that, indeed, the safety of the world appears in jeopardy. But even while all this was occurring, Parvati was standing off to the side watching. Just as the avatars can have one consciousness inhabiting several bodies, aspects of the great feminine such as Kali, too, can divide herself into the more reasonable Parvati, who in this context really serves as Kali's conscience, ever-present to keep things from going too far. If Kali and Shiva are the pot spinning wildly on the potter's wheel, Parvati is the potter's protective hand inside the spinning pot, ensuring that no harm comes.

In some of the previously referred to works called the tantras (treatises on the various paths to power and attainment including spiritual liberation), Kali is represented as supreme power. In the *Nirvana Tantra*, Brahma, Vishnu, and Shiva are said to rise from her like bubbles from the sea. Both the *Piccila Tantra* and the

Nigama Kalpataru proclaim that Kali's mantras are the most potent of all. It is true that every scripture declares that the subject of its writing embodies the supreme power, but there is wide agreement among a cross-section of teachings that the mystic fifteen-syllabled mantra of Kali, a form of which appears at the end of this chapter, is among a handful of the most powerful mantras of all.

The pursuit of Kali as a personal power to be invoked by anyone is a concept found in a study of a class of tantric texts that have sometimes been called "the left-hand path." It is here that tantra is misunderstood even in modern times. Students following the left-hand path are led by their teacher or guru to partake of forbidden things, namely wine, meat, fish, parched grain (which some have interpreted to mean a hallucinatory substance of some sort), and promiscuous sex. Here, Kali is the essence of everything that is forbidden, and her image is used as a focus to attain a transformation in a unity of opposites: unity of the sacred and the profane, of right and wrong, of virtue and dishonor. In the classical practice of the left-hand path, Kali is the dark and formless nature of the universe within which beings and planets wander. The gods are no more than the water collected in the hoofprint of a passing cow, while Kali is the ocean itself. All else, even the masculine trilogy of Brahma, Vishnu, and Shiva, is incidental.

Unfortunately, today, these higher-minded spiritual objectives of the left-hand path have given way to wanton behavior masking as acceptable religious practice. The acts themselves have become the central focus, and transcendence has been lost or forgotten altogether. Practices of those on the left-hand path have degenerated to a mostly sexually oriented yoga that produces momentary pleasure very far from the transformation that is the goal of any serious spiritual practice.

The Mantras of Kali

There are two mantras of Kali that I will present for your use in this chapter. Both are quite powerful. When stuck in an odd situation on the East Coast, while attempting to move to the West Coast, I used the first mantra below with great effect to extricate myself from the difficulty.

My contract as consultant to a public service foundation in Washington, D.C., was finished and other income sources on the East Coast dried up as a new political party took power in the nation's capital. At her suggestion, we decided to move to Los Angeles, the home of my new bride Margalo. Funds we were planning to use to move our family west were supposedly being released to us from where they were held on that coast, so we gave notice to our landlord and packed boxes for the move. A week before our departure date, an unexpected turn of events blocked access to the funds we had expected from California. We were suddenly stuck with no place to live and a house full of stuff packed in boxes. Luckily, our wonderful friend Mirabai offered to let us move into her house in suburban Virginia. Margalo and I and our two children shared a house with Mirabai, her husband, and her three children. It was cramped, but a great blessing. We stashed our boxes in storage and waited.

Fortunate though we were to have a refuge, we were stymied as to what to do next. After meditating on the issue, my intuition suggested a forty-day Kali mantra discipline.

In another part of my professional life, I was executive vice president of a multiethnic corporation that had applied for the last available television station license in Washington, D.C. Principals of our company had extensive experience in broadcasting and we were well regarded and ultimately aided by one of the top ten telecommunication law firms in the nation's capital. Although their legal expertise ran up a bill of hundreds of thousands of dollars, the firm provided all services needed for license filing to the FCC without taking a penny in advance. They were sure we would get the television station license, and said they would take their fees once the hearings before the FCC were over and the license had been granted. The dollar value of such a license is quite high; my stock alone was estimated at over $3 million.

I admit that my ego was heavily invested in this whole venture. I knew my ship was coming in. I had expertise in both commercial and public television, had worked hard, and was fortunate to have very skilled business associates.

Shortly after completing the discipline to Kali, I received a phone call from a minor shareholder in our television corporation. He had heard that I was in a fix and offered to buy a block of corporate shares from my portion of stock . . . for pennies on the dollar. He offered me a couple of dollars per share, although initial value was pegged at five times that value. After licensing, their value would be ten times that. I squirmed.

Kali had responded to my supplications through the mantra discipline, but at a price. I would have to accept a great loss, on paper, to get the money to move west. My ego squealed and groused. Here I had worked hard for so many years to achieve this goal that was nearly in sight, and now a big chunk was being taken from me. I was not very grateful, but I accepted Kali's grace in the form of the investor's offer and sold him a chunk of stock, complaining the whole time.

We subsequently completed our move to Los Angeles. In the meantime, the corporation waited for the FCC to rule. In 1983, the decision came down and we had won. We were ecstatic . . . until an appeal was filed by another group. The appeals process through the administrative law judge, a subsequent three-judge panel, the full FCC, and a federal appeals court was not resolved until 1990, and we lost. Another group was awarded the license and my stock was now worthless.

Kali had helped, but I had to confront and surrender a piece of my ego in the process. In the end, owning a piece of a television station was not part of my karma. I had to submit to the will of the divine, although not at all gracefully. I had to let go of something to which I was very attached. From an objective standpoint, Kali's grace was extremely compassionate, even if it was painful. She allowed me to begin the process of letting go of the television station long before the appeals process began. When we lost each appeal, I found I was prepared because I had been forced to begin detaching myself years before. Even though Kali's grace was thorough and complete, I didn't care for parts of it at all while it was taking place. This is often the way Kali works.

General Kali Mantra for Relief from Difficult Circumstances

This mantra can be used to bring one very quickly into balance or alignment with regard to a specific situation. The results can be dramatic and even unpleasant, even if they are ultimately the most compassionate. For instance, if you are having problems with a relationship and you use this Kali mantra to invoke her help with the problem, the relationship may end abruptly, even though this is not the outcome you desired. Conversely, a marriage possibility could develop much more quickly from a relationship than you might have desired or felt ready for. Whatever the issue, Kali gets right to the point and lets your ego attachments fall where they may. She is concerned with whatever will be the most beneficial outcome for you from a karmic standpoint, period.

1. **Om Klim Kalika-yei Namaha**
[Om Kleem Kah-lee-kah-yea Nahm-ah-hah]

"Om and salutations. I attract she who is dark and powerful."

Spiritual Evolution Mantra That Is Quick, Powerful, and Unyielding

There is also a longer form of the above mantra that relates to Kali as the destroyer of negative ego on the one hand, and the provider of a very fast route to spiritual liberation on the other. Although you might look for a long time, it would be difficult for you to discover this mantra, usually referred to simply and mysteriously as the Great Fifteen-Syllable Mantra. If you decide to work with this mantra, please have extra patience with yourself. Because it can work quickly, it may also cause some turmoil in your daily life.

The mantra will bring to the surface aspects of our ego that we have decided are "OK." We all become comfortable with ourselves in certain contexts. We know who we are, make allowances for our aberrant behavior, and fool ourselves that we are trying hard and doing the best we can. But if those internal qualities are truly not beneficial to us, this mantra will begin to eradicate even those characteristics we may have decided are "OK," and want to keep. If we are determined to hold on to parts of ourselves that are based on a deluded sense of satisfaction, particularly if our behavior is less than ideal, then Kali will come to our aid with a stainless-steel, scalpel-like precision.

When we invoke Kali through this mantra, we are saying, "I want true spiritual advancement by the most powerful and direct route, the consequences to my ego notwithstanding." So if you pick this route, its only fair that you know what you are in for. It will be intense, possibly unnerving, probably uncomfortable, certainly disruptive to one or more aspects of your mundane life, and also very effective in a short amount of time.

**2. Om Hrim Shreem Klim Adya Kalika Param
Eshwari Swaha**
[Om Hreem Shreem Kleem Ahd-yah Kah-lee-kah
Pah-rahm Ehsh-wah-ree Swah-hah]
"Om and salutations to She who is the first one, dark
within her own reality, the supreme primordial feminine,
who cuts through illusion to the unabridged truth of
existence."

7

Lalita

The Great Feminine with a Thousand Powers

I don't think it is an overstatement to say that all the great teachers of yoga, and popular gurus who have come to the West, have had a direct and powerful relationship to, and with, the Great Feminine principle. Paramahansa Yogananda spoke reverently of his beloved Divine Mother to whom he prayed when in difficulty and who he claimed healed him of a terrible leg problem just before a speaking engagement. Paramahansa Ramakrishna, utterly devoted to his Mother Kali, had a profound experience with her when he and Sarada Devi were married. Even though Sarada Devi was still a young girl and he a grown man, the wedding ceremony was performed according to tradition. At the conclusion, he placed her on a table and performed puja to her as Divine Mother, whereupon they flew into a sublime state together. In one of his poems, the great sage of Pondicherry, Sri Aurobindo, said of the Great Feminine that "She is the Divine Matrix to whom all of nature dumbly calls." Paramahansa Muktananda was a Shaivite, or worshiper of the masculine Shiva principle. But to him, Shakti and Shiva are manifestations of each other as the same entity. When Muktananda initiated people, he did so by Shaktipat Diksha: the transfer of shakti.

These are but a few of the sages and gurus known in the West who revered the Great Feminine. While some people may already be familiar with these teachers, it seems not to have resonated properly in the Western, nonacademic mind (contemporary scholars, however, have well understood and chronicled the power of the Great Feminine) that the Great Feminine holds the key to our spiritual advancement and even liberation itself. This may be due to our Western orientation to God the Father.

I would like to return here to an idea presented in an earlier part of this book, namely the idea of a feminine power cell that sits at the base of the human spine in the *Muladhara* chakra. Seeming to sleep and without using even a hundred-thousandth part of the energy dormant within her, She provides all the power for life's activities, both autonomic and conscious. Often called simply Divine Mother, it is our shakti that releases within us the energy and influence of the planets in our lives as recorded in our astrological chart. Like a cosmic engine, those orbs circulate in the solar system, interact with one another, and send out their multiple vibrations. As these subtle vibrations strike our bodies at birth and then continuously throughout our lives, it is our shakti that activates their power within, causing events and circumstances to whirl around us as occurrences in daily life.

It is also our shakti that causes great waves of thought and emotion to manifest as our *samsaras*, those mental and emotional tendencies with which we enter life. And it is she who knows how long the span of a given incarnation will last. Desiring more time to complete his work, it was Divine Mother whom Paramahansa Yogananda entreated, sensing the end of his life drawing near. He desired just a few more years to finish his life's work, and it was Divine Mother, his actively powerful benevolent shakti, who granted his wish.

In our exploration of the Great Feminine, we have met Saraswati, the consort of Brahma, who is the Divine Word, representing the power of speech in such a dimension and capability that the universe can emerge from it. She is a part of Narayana and joins with Vishnu to help lead souls back to their ultimate divine source and spiritual destiny. We have encountered Durga and Kali, the unleashed fury of the Great Feminine who protects us while purifying our motives until they are pristine enough to behold her directly. While she destroys those negative forces that would enslave the pious ones, she also tenderly guards and blesses the innocent.

Now we come to Lalita—She of a thousand names and powers. Although the word *thousand* is used, it is symbolic of and synonymous with numberless, countless.

Lalita is the hidden feminine who provides a route to tremendous attainment in this life. Protected from common view, she is little written or talked about except among small groups of seekers, usually at remote monasteries or through a very few organizations that have stumbled upon the depth of what is contained in the verses dedicated to her: *The Lalita Sahasranama.*

This great work, which has become a scripture in its own right, comprises the second half of *The Brahmananda Purana*, of which there are several versions. The most popular and accessible version takes the form of a conversation between Sage Hayagriva and his student and great disciple Sage Agastya. Because the oral history of how these powers came down to the current era is emphasized rather than the story of the goddess herself, the discussion of Lalita that follows will be a bit different from the stories in the previous chapters.

In the *Mahabharata*, originating well over five thousand years ago according to the oral tradition in India, it is stated that every form of knowledge has its source in one of the many forms of

Bhagavan Vishnu. The *Mahabharata* claims, unequivocally, that because Sage Hayagriva is a direct emanation of Vishnu (clearly
indicated as such in many Puranic sources), his teachings concerning the most powerful paths to liberation are to be very seri-
ously studied. Hayagriva was often called the horse-faced one.
This unusual diminutive is easily understood when one considers
that many Indian teachers question whether he was human in the
same sense that you and I are, or from some other place wearing
a semi-human disguise, as many of the avatars of Vishnu are reputed to be.

In any case, Hayagriva taught the secret doctrine of Sri Vidya,
the knowledge of the Great Feminine and various practices relating to it. Hayagriva's knowledge of the laws and operational procedures of the cosmos, the essence of Sri Vidya, sometimes called
Brahma Vidya, is partially transmitted through the *Lalita Sahasranama*. This scripture has come down to us today only because it
stands upon a stable, proverbial three-legged stool: the divine
power of Sage Hayagriva, the unusual competence of his discipline Agastya, and the might of Divine Mother herself. After
teaching the secrets of Sri Vidya or divine knowledge to his great
disciple, Hayagriva then retired to a remote place for a life of
contemplation and meditation.

The Story of Sage Agastya

While he was still a student, Agastya realized that there was
one final piece needed for his divine education that he had not
yet received: the power of the Great Feminine, Lalita. Taking into
consideration the nature of his teacher and his own attainments,
Agastya thought: "Could the lack of my receiving this precious
teaching be a conscious omission by Hayagriva? Or could it be

that the Master thought me unsuitable to learn? Certainly a great guru will not be lax toward a genuine discipline? What reason could there be for him to keep back a part of the teaching? Have I not real desire to learn? Have I not served my guru with deep reverence?"

Agastya came to the conclusion that he may be unfit to learn the missing piece, so he finally asked Hayagriva the reason for the neglect. The spiritual preceptor Hayagriva spoke with delight and compassion. "Listen to me attentively. Well have I not given you the thousand names of Sri Lalita Ambika, as it is a guarded secret. Now that you are asking for it with great devotion, I am going to give it to you. Even if the subject is not meant for open teaching, it should definitely be taught by a teacher to a fit and devoted discipline. In your time you, too, should not give this holy gift to anyone who has no spiritual honor or who is wily and impure, has no respect for the true spiritual teacher, or is bereft of devotion to Divine Mother. A wise teacher is averse to teach a person who does not ask for instruction. But he may impart it to deserving ones who have genuine faith in the teacher and great interest in learning this teaching.

"There may even be ones who have great faith and devotion of this kind, but have no confidence to ask the teacher. Such people may also be taught graciously, even without their praying or asking for it. Religious faith, loving adoration, humble questioning, and moral purity make one eligible for seeking such precious matters."

Pausing to see that Agastya had assimilated what he had said, Hayagriva continued. "Long ago [and his "long ago" was from a perspective of several thousand years before our time], Lalita Ambika [another name for Durga or Parvati] summoned for the benefit of her devotees the various goddesses of speech, divine utterance and sacred observances, manifestation and other sacred abilities related to The Word. She said to them, 'You all have diverse powers of speech through my Grace, and you are appropriate for conferring them upon my devotees. You know the secret of my *Sri Yantra* (sacred design of the universe sometimes called the *Sri Chakra*) and are extremely devoted to my name. Therefore, I now order you to produce a hymn about me. Let it include my thousand names and be of such quality that by the recitation of it my devotees receive my favors without delay.' "

Hayagriva continued, "Divine Mother was seated upon her throne of universal sovereignty, which provided a great opportunity for her to be propitiated and her interests served. The gods came in indescribable number: Brahma and Saraswati, Narayana and Lakshmi, Rudra and Gauri, divine shaktis (or embodied powers), holy sages, and celestials also came such as Brahmarishi Vishwamitra, Siddha Yogis and Saptarishis Narada, Sanaka and the rest. All endlessly came before her." Finally, those divine feminine ones, *devies*, who had heard her command came before her and with folded hands delivered the *Lalita Sahasranama* that we have with us today. She was overwhelmingly pleased at their performance and the entire assembly was filled with joy, for it was a perfect piece of sacred literature, pregnant with mystic power and spiritual wisdom. Over the intervening millennia, it has also come to be esoterically called the *Rahasya Nama*, or the scripture of mysterious secret names.

The *Brahmananda Purana* proclaims, "Recitation of even one of these thousand names is said to have more merit than taking a bath in the Ganges, performing various austerities, or giving to Brahmins. All sins, even grave ones, committed by one who says the full thousand names, will be washed away by a single recitation of these names. There is no evil act that cannot be rectified by chanting these thousand names with devotion on a regular basis. To look for another source to erase sins would be like going to a snowy mountain to escape the cold."

These grand forms of praise help to motivate us as seekers after truth. It is for our benefit, spiritual and material, that these potent formulas, so powerful in stimulating the chakras and the kundalini, have been made available to us. The recitation of the full complement of mantras rapidly removes all manner of karma. But recitation of even one or two is an extremely powerful way to effect changes in our spiritual and material circumstances. In *Healing Mantras*, I told the story of the bank security guard who changed the way he was perceived by women after less than twenty-five hours of chanting a single mantra from this scripture. It is mantra number one, given at the end of this chapter.

It is said that in Sage Agastya were combined stupendous powers, unparalleled disciplines, and vast, profound learning. And because of his spiritual standing and great knowledge, there came a time when he was called upon to help in turning the cosmic wheel, so to speak. . . .

Sage Agastya, Favorite of Shiva and Parvati

Sage Agastya's home was in the Himalayan Mountains. Here with his elevated spouse, Lopamudra (who shared his consciousness), he established a place to contemplate the higher purposes of life. The heights of the mountains and inaccessibility of their hermitage made for just the kind of depth of existence Agastya desired. One day when he dived deep into his usual meditative state, Lord Shiva appeared to him and asked a favor. He requested that Agastya move his residence from Mount Kailas in northern India/Tibet to the southern portion of the Indian subcontinent.

Offering no substantial reason, Shiva asked Agastya if he would be willing to consider such a move. Now, Agastya knew that to see Shiva in meditation was a great blessing. Thus, he did not hesitate for even one moment before he assented to Shiva's request, even though he knew he would miss the icy silence of the Himalayas. He also knew that Lopamudra would be much happier in the south. So gathering their meager supply of belongings and taking with him the scriptures explaining the powers of Lalita, given to him by Hayagriva, Agastya and Lopamudra traveled to the south and made their abode in the steaming forests of southern India. Then came a bit of an annoyance.

Shiva was soon to be wed to Parvati, but Agastya, now far removed from the Himalayas, was unable to attend the grand ceremony. In fact, surprisingly, he and Lopamudra had not even received an invitation. As he sat in meditation two days before the scheduled marriage, a feeling of loss came over him. However, he resolutely pushed the feeling away, thanked the divine for his many blessings, and sank deeper into his meditation. Nearing the edge of his ability to remain conscious of himself as an individual being in the universe, while still in the ever-deepening throes of bliss, Agastya suddenly saw a brilliant ball of light in the center of his meditative sight. Approaching with increasing speed and brightness, it soon occupied one-third of his entire field of vision. Finally, it came to a stop and dissolved into the supple and beguiling form of young Parvati.

Smiling at him with a beatific radiance, she spoke to him. "Agastya, Shiva and I are about to marry. Yet I do not find you or Lopamudra among the guests waiting to march in the wedding party. Are you so busy with meditation that you cannot spare us a day or even a few hours?"

With joined palms in his mind's eye, Agastya replied with great reverence. "Holy Mother, did your beloved Shiva not tell you? We have moved to the southern portion of the continent. Thus, we are nowhere near you. It would take six months to reach you and then the same to return again. I must also tell you that we did not receive an invitation to attend your wedding. How would it serve if one of us were to arrive, uninvited, like a thistle plant among beautiful flowers?"

Parvati threw back her head laughing, sending dark ringlets of shiny, silken hair cascading over her back, down her embroidered red sari. "Agastya, what are we to do with you? Wherever I am, you are always welcome. And Shiva, himself, asked where you were, saying his celebration would not be complete without your presence. Lopamudra, the very epitome of your own nature with all its power and humility, is always welcome no matter what the occasion."

If it were possible to turn a pink, embarrassed color in meditation, Agastya would surely have done so. "Surely Shiva must know that it is by his request that we have come all this way to the south. Being the very wellspring of consciousness, he cannot have forgotten." Although rock solid in his meditative pose, Agastya felt like squirming out of sheer disbelief.

"No, great sage, Shiva has not forgotten. In fact, I have just been playing with you a bit. It was he who asked me to come and grant you the favor that is forthcoming."

"What favor is that?" replied Agastya. "I have asked for nothing."

"Oh, we know that," said Parvati, "but it is no exaggeration that our wedding would be incomplete without your presence, so by my power you will see everything just as if you were present. I will construct for you a proxy body for your consciousness. It will contain senses for you to see, hear, and smell everything about the ceremony and procession. If you wish, I will also make that body ambulatory so that you may stroll with us in the first group of sages, just behind where we will be walking. Would you like that, Agastya?" Parvati's eyes poured forth mirth and joy all mixed together.

Agastya's heart swelled with gratitude and the warmth of his body reached his consciousness even in deep meditation. "Words cannot be found to state how joyfully I accept your invitation in all of its aspects," Agastya said with reverence. "To be there and walk with you is more than I ever could have hoped for. What must I do to prepare? And what about Lopamudra?"

"You need do nothing at all," replied Parvati. "Just sit in meditation starting at dawn the day after tomorrow, and leave everything to me. As for Lopamudra, I have asked her to assist my parents in the preparations for the ceremony, I hope you don't mind. After I asked her, she immediately agreed and has already left." With those final words, she dissolved once more into a ball of light and rapidly receded into the distance. Agastya was alone as before, seated for his usual dawn meditation. Pulling a smooth woolen shawl over his shoulders, he quickly scanned the room of their humble cottage to ensure that he had left no pot cooking, or window flap open with rain approaching. No, everything was in good order. Without further delay, Agastya settled into his customary seat and began to withdraw energy from his senses, his limbs, and the rest of his body. The energy flowed back into his spine and he began to focus it upward toward his brain. After no more than ten minutes Agastya entered a deep state.

"Oh, you are here right on schedule, I see." Parvati's brilliant form glided into view from his peripheral vision on the left side. "Good. Come, follow me." She floated up toward what would have been the top of his head in his mind's eye.

With a slight strain, Agastya tried to lift himself up from inside but could not seem to dislodge himself from his body. Pausing in her flight, Parvati wordlessly returned and, reaching down, lifted him effortlessly. Agastya felt himself detach from his body and lift out of it smoothly. With a glancing smile over her shoulder, Parvati zipped away into the dark azure morning, as the sun was preparing to arrive for the day. With an almost giddy sense of freedom, Agastya followed her up and out of his and Lopamudra's hidden hermitage. Gaining incredible speed, they soon left the forest area and sped due north. In no time at all, the Himalayas appeared in the distance, like gigantic soldiers guarding the way into their huge valleys. A left turn here, a veer to the right there, and Mount Kailas was in sight.

Now Parvati slowed and deftly maneuvered them toward a small clearing on the north side of Kailas, finally landing a hundred paces from the cottage she and Shiva shared. Motioning to a smaller hut off to the side, Parvati pulled Agastya by the hand until they reached the hut where she opened the door. There, sitting in complete stillness was a body that looked exactly like Agastya. It did not breathe, nor move even a hair on its arm, looking almost waxen. With a small flourish, Parvati pulled Agastya around so that his back faced the lifeless form, then she pushed him backward so that he literally fell into it.

For a second he was disoriented, but then his consciousness filtered into the form, and he inhabited it completely. He opened his eyes and saw Parvati positively beaming back at him. "Shiva will be so pleased!" she said.

Agastya found that his arms and legs behaved quite normally. Realizing that the body would respond in every way like the one he left in the south, Agastya rose to his feet and strode toward the door leading to the outside. As he opened the door, a shaft of sunlight reflecting off the glacier sheet in the distance hit him full in the face. Agastya had gone only ten paces from the door to the hut when Shiva came around the corner grinning so broadly that the cobra around his neck had to slightly rearrange itself.

"Don't mind my Naga friend here," said Shiva. "He insists on joining me in meditation, even if I sit for only a few minutes. I was just finishing up when you arrived. Here, come for some tea." Shiva gestured toward his small house just as Parvati stuck her head out the door and shouted for them to come and get a fresh cup of tea. Agastya noted that Shiva and Parvati were completely joined in consciousness, as one being inhabiting two bodies.

After tea, Shiva and Parvati began to discuss plans for the next three days of the wedding. Once they left here, the couple explained, there would be little time to speak for the next three days. All of a sudden, Agastya realized he had no gift for the couple. Not one thing. He tried to hide his sudden sickening realization, but his face utterly betrayed him. With wide eyes, Parvati addressed the sage. "What has happened, O jewel of Shiva's mind? You look like someone has just died."

Reflecting for less time than a flea takes in deciding which way to jump, Shiva arrived at the heart of Agastya's problem. "Oh-h-h-h, I see," he muttered. Sitting completely silent for just a moment, Shiva spoke again, this time to Parvati. "O mother of all that is, when are Rama and Sita due to appear on Earth?"

Parvati stared vacantly off into space for less than a second, then replied, "They will arrive in another thousand years, give or take, why?" Answering her own question, she spoke again. "Oh, yes, I see what you are driving at." She went over and kissed Shiva on the top of his head and set the tray down. The cobra, still hanging around Shiva's neck, almost seemed to purr in response.

Shiva spoke in gentle tones to Agastya. "I know that you were startled by your sudden ability to attend the wedding. Therefore your source of embarrassment: no gift for the bride and groom. It is true that we have everything we will ever need, but you can satisfy your desire to give us something if you will do a favor I have to ask of you. It is no small thing."

Agastya breathed a sigh of relief. A crack had appeared in the wall of his dilemma. "I will be only too happy to oblige whatever you ask." He looked at and addressed Parvati. "I would only hope that you will desire this favor as much as Shiva."

Parvati jumped in. "Oh, believe me, I want this very much. Rama will . . . sorry, you don't even know what the favor is yet. . . ."

Shiva announced the favor they requested. "The gift I want from you is to share what your great teacher, Sage Hayagriva, has taught to you about the Great Feminine with the Avatar Rama who will appear in a thousand years or so. Now, I know you are wondering how you will still be around at that time, but that is a small matter. Parvati and I can arrange that with very little trouble. What I want is that you teach the young Rama mantras that are found in the *Lalita Sahasranama*. He will need to know such things in his contest with the evil Ravana."

"I have never met nor even heard of this Rama fellow," replied Agastya pensively. "I have no desire to dishonor my teacher, Hayagriva. Nor do I mean you any disrespect. But these matters are not casually taught." Sage Agastya sat in an ever-increasing stewlike simmer.

"However much I agree, I confess that the reason I asked you to move to the southern part of India has to do with the arrival of Sita and Rama in the next millennium." Shiva absently played with the Naga around his neck. "The knowledge you now have comes from Vishnu, via Hayagriva, an aspect of Vishnu. Rama and Sita will be avatars of Vishnu and Lakshmi, respectively. Thus, you will do no harm whatsoever in giving to Vishnu, in the form of Rama, that which originally came from him anyway. In fact, you will be greatly aiding dharma, since Rama must defeat the cunning and powerful Ravana in order to restore righteousness to human affairs once again."

Agastya was not yet satisfied. "Not only do I not know who Rama is, I have no idea who this fellow Ravana is you have referred to. Nor Sita either, for that matter. And why should any knowledge I might have be useful to any avatar? They come into embodiment with everything they could possibly need."

Parvati smiled again with that effulgent radiance that threatened to instantly reduce the size of a hundred nearby glaciers. With infinite tenderness and patience, she spoke to Agastya. "O noble object of Lopamudra's undying love and affection, I shall explain to you that which you have so artfully requested. It is certainly true the avatars of Vishnu come into embodiment with whatever they need to accomplish their purpose. But it is also true that they structure a drama around events that will allow them to help and bless as many people as possible. Knowing this, please accede to our request, and fulfill your desire to give us something for our formal union. Any contact you have with the coming Avatar Rama will only be a great blessing to you anyway. Come, quickly agree before the tea gets cold and I must run and heat it up once more."

Agastya had no more questions. He bowed his head and spoke softly, "I will do as you request. I know that it is not possible for one such as you to ask anything improper, so even though I have no knowledge of this Rama fellow, if he presents himself to me, I will teach him. But please know that I will clearly state that it is by your grace and through no merit of my own that this teaching comes to him."

Parvati spoke. "Now that that's settled, I must make ready to leave. You two can continue in *satsang* [divine discussion] for a little while. Then we must take flight to my parents' home. We will take you to where Lopamudra is staying, and then not see you until the procession." Turning away satisfied and happy in every way, Parvati glided back to their cottage while Shiva and Agastya discussed some of the finer points of self-conscious existence.

The wedding took place on a grand scale, and Lopamudra and Agastya marched with the other exalted sages just a few paces behind Shiva and Parvati. A divinely wonderful time was had by all, and then it was over. Parvati helped Agastya and Lopamudra return home, and then with a cheery wave she left to be with Shiva on Kailas.

For many years Agastya stayed at the hermitage and taught students at various levels of development. At certain odd times, he and Lopamudra would retire for the night, only to find in the morning that a hundred years or more had passed. Yet even at these times, Agastya found that his fame as a spiritual teacher remained undiminished. New batches of students would appear and be taught various spiritual mysteries, although only a handful would ever receive the teachings pertaining to the *Lalita Sahasranama*.

As Parvati had said, about a thousand years later, Rama was finally born, and the drama of his life began to unfold. As part of that drama, Rama was required to wander in the forests of south India for fourteen years. During these travels, Rama heard about the hermitage of Sage Agastya and eventually visited him there to pay homage to the great sage and his wisdom, Lopamudra.

As part of his homage to Rama, Agastya gave Rama a great bow to use in battle. Esoterically, the bow is knowledge of how to use any mantra. The arrows that fly from the bow are the mantras themselves. Agastya also taught Rama the holy hymn called the *Aditya Hridaya* that concerns the creative power and nature of the flame with many names burning in the sacred heart, that many call Narayana, some call Lakshmi, and a few call Lalita. Finally, he taught Rama the secrets of Sri Vidya through the *Lalita Sahasranama*. With this piece of knowledge, Rama was ready to assume the full mantle of his authority as an avatar. Thankful for the assistance of Agastya and Lopamudra, Rama blessed them with *mukti*, or spiritual liberation. Shiva and Parvati had known that Rama would bestow this jewel upon them, but they wanted to keep it a surprise, otherwise where's the fun?

A Few Loose Ends

It was Agastya's purity of consciousness that allowed him supreme access to the Great Feminine. So complete was this purity that he did not need to travel anywhere with his physical body. He could go anywhere at any time, mentally. If this is the case, then why did he and Lopamudra move, physically, to the south? They did so specifically to aid the Avatar Rama, who was due to appear in the future. The opportunity to be of use to the Avatar Rama and thereby be granted liberation was a gift of Shiva and Parvati to Sage Agastya and Lopamudra. After all, the divine knowledge pertaining to the Great Feminine had originally come from Vishnu and Lakshmi in the first place. Oh, what a tangled web of divine grace these celestials weave!

Mantras and More

The thousand Lalita mantras are part of an eight-hour feminine ceremony I conduct at various venues during the year. This ceremony can help to amplify and anchor any spiritual discipline involving mantra. The very nature and intensity of a daylong ceremony of this type also clears away negativity that may have become lodged deep within during the course of daily life. So it is both cleansing and empowering.

I will provide you with a few of the mantras, their meaning, and what they can do for you. But first, we must touch upon the Sri Yantra (diagram), also called Sri Chakra, a great mystical symbol that is said to provide access to the powers of the activities of the universe.

Sri Chakra—the Power of the Universe

As complex as the Kabbalistic Tree of Life, and symbolizing the very essence of the Great Feminine, is a mystical diagram called the Sri Yantra that illustrates and details the Sri Chakra, or Wheel of Splendor, or Her Wheel. Chakra, you will recall, means wheel, but here the "wheel" is the universe itself. The honorific "Sri" is a word commonly used as an address of great reverence reserved for those who are spiritually very advanced. What is not well known is that the honor of this title lies in the fact that "Sri" refers to the Great Feminine, the great all-pervading power. Using this title when referring to an individual implies that the feminine power is awake and functioning in the individual, something not often the case today for those upon whom this honorific is bestowed.

But in the Sri Chakra, the word *Sri* is meant to convey the idea that the very power of the elements that compose the universe— that is, all the energy that composes all matter (remember, matter equals energy in patterns of configuration in Eastern thought) as well as the finished product—is feminine in nature.

Of course, there is a story behind this that links the Sri Chakra to Lalita. Briefly, in an effort to repel the evil advances of the demon king Bhanda, the celestial leader Indra built an altar on the banks of the Bhagairathi River in the foothills of the Himalayas. There he intended to perform a fire ceremony invoking the Supreme Power, Para Shakti. But from the middle of the altar, the Sri Chakra magically and resplendently appeared, and from the center of this chakra, Lalita herself emerged. She took on the evil Bhanda and his demon forces, ultimately killing the demon king and restoring peace to the universe. Therefore, to meditate on the

Sri Chakra is said to be the equivalent of contemplating all aspects of the cosmos in a single, glorious, all-encompassing symbol. The Sri Chakra is an impersonal representation, while Lalita is a personal, anthropomorphized one.

The Sri Chakra is a complex mandala composed of nine overlapping triangles. Although some sources actually reverse this construction, most commonly four triangles (representing aspects of consciousness) point upward, and five (representing the five elements) point downward. To fully explain this wonder is frankly beyond the scope of this book. It's no exaggeration to say that one could spend many years, even a lifetime, studying and meditating to fathom and integrate the intricacies and mysteries of the Sri Chakra and Sri Lalita. Here is just the briefest overview to give you a taste.

The four triangles pointing upward are:

Chitta—raw mind stuff
Manas—functioning mind
Buddhi—intellect—that aspect of mind where great ideas are born, perceived, or entered into from some other place of origin
Ahamkara—ego born of mind

One or more of these elements can be used to describe any aspect or activity of the human mind. Thus, any evolving state is contained within these concepts, even if the state of consciousness is one far in the future that exists in us now only as a seed. Such seeds may be thought of as the acorn of our potential consciousness's oak. Any possible state the human mind can attain is implicit within this pattern, even the potential to transcend matter. The diagram implies that these states are well understood and attainable.

The five triangles pointing downward, called Pancha Maha Bhuta (the five great elements) in Sanskrit, stand for:

Earth
Water
Fire
Air
Ether

These elements, also identified and considered by the ancient Greeks, cover any and all aspects of our material creation. Four of these elements are familiar to us, while the fifth, ether, is a bit more mysterious. This element, however, is the gateway to the knowledge of the universe that is stored in nonphysical reality and accessible only through mind. Unlimited by time or space, it is this realm that many great psychics tap into for information unavailable by the usual mundane means.

Perhaps you have noticed that we have, in the four upward triangles, the idea of the masculine, consciousness, and in the five downward-pointing triangles the idea of feminine energy. Indeed, the four aspects of consciousness are often referred to as "the fires" and the five elements of nature are referred to as the "shaktis." From the fivefold shakti comes creation, and from the fourfold fires comes dissolution at the end of time in any created universe.

At the center of the Sri Chakra are three more points of interest:

Bindhu—the individual self
Nada—the principle of sound
Kala—light rays, which define time

One is red, symbolizing the ovum; one white, symbolizing the sperm; and one is mixed, the union of shiva and shakti, consciousness and energy.

The Sri Chakra is a grand synthesis of time, space, and humankind. To describe and explain the various levels and elements would take its own book. If the subject fascinates you, I highly encourage independent study.

There is a specific mantra associated with the Sri Chakra symbol that can activate the kundalini in an exceedingly powerful way and that has the attributes of being both powerful and safe. Number one below is one of the thousand powers contained in the *Lalita Sahasranama*.

To Invoke the Primal Creative Power of the Universe

This mantra will gently and powerfully activate Kriya Shakti. Indra states in his hymn of praise to Lakshmi, called the *Maha Lakshmi Astakam*, that although she is the spouse of Vishnu, she is also the power of Shiva manifesting through Parvati. As such, when the celestials and demons churned the ocean of consciousness in search of the Nectar of Immortality (see Chapter 3), it was the great Kriya Shakti of Lakshmi they invoked. So powerful were those efforts, originally recommended by Shiva, that the physical universe was created and Lakshmi made her appearance to take her part in the divine drama.

1. Om Shrim Shriyei Namaha
[Om Shreem Shree-yei Nahm-ah-hah]
"Om and salutations to the creative abundance that is the very form of this universe."

Foundation Mantra for Lalita

Sage Hayagriva gave this foundation mantra for common use to attain knowledge, which can be accumulated as a tangible force, to be subsequently applied to almost any situation.

2. Om Eim Klim Sau Sau Klim Eim
[Om I'm Kleem Saw Saw Kleem I'm]

Consisting entirely of seed syllables, this mantra can greatly help to improve concentration and attract shakti to the four elements of mind/consciousness described above.

For Neutralizing, or "Forgiving," Negative Acts Resulting in Less Than Good Karma

3. Om Papa Nashinyei Namaha
[Om Pah-pah Nahsh-een-yei Nah-mah-hah]
"Salutations to She who destroys sins completely by the use of mantra formulas."

General Mantra for Fulfilling Desires

The best way to use this mantra is to concentrate on the desired object or conditions, while chanting the mantra.

4. Om Kama Dayinyei Namaha
[Om Kah-mah Dah-een-yei Nah-mah-hah]
"Salutation to She who is compassion itself."

General Mantra to Rid the Mind and Body of Depression

By saying this mantra, you are stimulating the kundalini shakti to provide the state inherent in the energy of the syllables. That energy is antithetical to the state of depression.

5. Om Bhoginyei Namaha
[Om Bhoh-geen-yei Nah-mah-hah]
"Salutations to She who has the experience of perpetual bliss."

General Mantra for Ridding the Mind of an Unwanted Desire

This mantra is best practiced with a preparatory step. First, remove the unwanted desire from your concentration. I know, this is like saying "Don't think about a duck." You weren't thinking about a duck before, but now you can't think about anything else. The basic idea is to frame your intention in advance, but then, when chanting your mantra, not to dwell on that intention, that desire from which you seek release.

6. Om Nishka Mayei Namaha
[Om Neesh-kah Mah-yei Nah-mah-ha]
"Salutations to She who is free from desires."

Festival of the Great Feminine

Worship of the Great Feminine takes place every Fall in India, where a festival called Navaratri is observed. Originally, a similar festival was held in honor of the Great Feminine at the beginning of each season, but over the last several hundred years it has come to be performed only around harvest time, the first nine days of autumn, calculated by the lunar calendar. Three days of chanting and pujas are dedicated to each of the feminine trinity: the first three belong to Lakshmi; days four through six are Saraswati's; and days seven, eight, and nine honor Durga. The festival ends on a tenth day with a grand ceremony called Vijaya Dasami, or "Victory of the Mother who serves all." Saluting all the goddesses, Vijaya Dasami is one of the most widely observed spiritual celebration days in India, cutting across many barriers of caste and creed.

Everyone desires the Divine Mother's blessing. Some seek abundance, while others seek to solve family problems pertaining to marriage or in-laws. Health concerns of one kind or another make up the prayers of millions, as well. Whatever the difficulty or desire, the grace of the Great Feminine is sought through this festival. It is very common during Navaratri to see people going about their daily lives with lips moving slightly as they quietly chant mantras to Durga, Lakshmi, or Saraswati.

Maha Shakti Puja

Interest in the Great Feminine has grown so rapidly over the last few years that I was inspired to put together a special eight-hour ceremony (including breaks and lunchtime) based on Lalita. Adding to her thousand names, I include the 108 names (called *Astotaras*) for Durga, Lakshmi, and Saraswati. We finally chant 1,324 names of Divine Mother and many verses and hymns (*shlokas*) for each of the goddesses.

The complete ceremony is composed of three parts, each of which builds upon the previous part. For about three hours, interspersed with breaks, the assembled group chants special mantras together. This is followed by the ceremonial bathing of the *murtis* (small symbolic statues of the goddesses), with each person participating according to her or his inclination to do so.

Contrary to the way things are done in India, where only puja sponsors participate in the ceremony, I offer each person who attends the option of participating. At the place in the ceremony where the ceremonial oblations are performed, I encourage those who wish to be involved in the ceremony to come forward and perform their own personal oblation to the Great Feminine, telling attendees, "If Mary is dear to you, feel that you are offering a ceremonial spiritual bathing to her. Or if Isis is revered, then offer oblations to her." And so forth. This kind of personal oblation by each person usually takes between thirty and sixty seconds. Then the individual returns to her or his seat for meditation and prayer while I continue chanting the sacred verses accompanied by a ringing bell. Since Margalo often performs this service with me, two powerful Tibetan bells accompany the many different verses and hymns to the goddesses over the next three hours.

Finally, we all gather around the symbols of the Great Feminine, and the chanting of the 1,324 names begins. As I complete each of the mantras, the group choruses the final *"Namaha"* and throws a grain of rice toward the murtis. This act symbolizes both a salutation to the goddess and an invocation of the named power within. When this is finished, we share fruit and a special sweet food prepared for the ceremony as an offering.

In the fall of 1999, I first announced that I was making this ceremony available, and within ten days three had been scheduled to take place during the next three months. One of the first organizations to schedule a Maha Shakti Puja (literally, ceremony invoking the power of the Great Feminine) was the Church of Truth in Pasadena, California. The minister wished to have her church imbued with the energy of the Great Feminine as soon as we reached 2000, so the ceremony was scheduled for January 2.

It is impossible to convey the various sensations, emotions, and the sense of power this ceremony can generate. It's honestly a case of "you have to be there" (and I do hope you will soon have the experience, if you have not already). Below is a handful of the mantra-powers taken from the *Lalita Sahasranama* that are chanted in the last part of the ceremony.

88. Om Mula Mantra'tmikayei Namaha
[Om Moo-lah Mahn-traht-mee-kah-yei Nahm-ah-hah]
"Om and salutations to She who is the power of the foundation feminine mantras."

96. Om Akulayei Namah
[Om Ah-koo-lah-yei Nahm-ah-hah]

"Om and salutations to She who, having risen to the thousand-petaled lotus at the top of the head, is referred to as 'akula,' having no perceivable genesis, lineage, or qualities whatsoever."

98. Om Muladhara'ik Nilayayei Namaha
[Om Moo-lah-dhah-rah-eek Nee-lah-yah-yei Nahm-ah-hah]
"Om and salutations to She who is the kundalini power residing in the Muladhara chakra at the base of the spine."

117. Om Bhakta Saubhagya Dayinyei Namaha
[Om Bhahk-tah Sauw-bhag-gyah Dah-yeen-yei Nahm-ah-hah]
"Om and salutations to She who compassionately gives qualities of herself to Her devotees, including illumination, glory, beauty, and other attributes making their future bright."

119. Om Bhakti Gamayei Namaha
[Om Bhahk-tee Gahm-ah-yei Nahm-ah-hah]
"Om and salutations to She who is reached through devotion and service."

121. Om Bhaya Pahayei Namaha
[Om Bhah-yah Pah-hah-yei Nahm-ah-hah]
"Om and salutations to She who removes fear by empowering with knowledge."

127. Om Sri Karayei Namaha
[Om Shree Kah-rah-yei Nahm-ah-hah]

"Om and salutations to She who became Lakshmi, the spouse of Vishnu."

149. Om Nitya Buddhayei Namaha
[Om Neet-yah Bood-hah-yei Nahm-ah-hah]
"Om and salutations to She who is the abode of Knowledge."

159. Om Mada Nashinyei Namaha
[Om Mah-dah Nash-een-yei Nahm-ah-hah]
"Om and salutations to She who eradicates arrogance."

191. Om Dukha Hantrayei Namaha
[Om Dook-hah Hahn-trah-yei Nahm-ah-hah]
"Om and salutations to She who eradicates the sorrows of this world."

200. Om Sarva Mangalayei Namaha
[Om Sahr-vah Mahn-gahl-ah-yei Nahm-ah-hah]
"Om and salutations to She who is all auspiciousness and gives the same to Her devotees."

204. Om Sarva Mantra Swarupinyei Namaha
[Om Sahr-vah Mahn-trah Swah-roop-een-yei Nahm-ah-hah]
"Om and salutations to She who is the ultimate form of all mantras and sacred formulas."

224. Om Maha Siddhayei Namaha
[Om Mah-hah Seed-hah-yei Nahm-ah-hah]
"Om and salutations to She who is the abode of spiritual abilities or powers and bestows them upon her devotees."

241. Om Charu Rupayei Namaha

[Om Chah-roo Roo-pah-yei Nahm-ah-hah]

"Om and salutations to She who embodies beauty and elegance."

256. Om Vishwa Rupayei Namaha

[Om Veesh-wah Roo-pah-yei Nahm-ah-hah]

"Om and salutations to She who is the form of the entire universe."

292. Om Purnayei Namaha

[Om Poor-nah-yei Nahm-ah-hah]

"Om and salutations to She who is complete, unified, and perfect, without limitation of any kind."

301. Om Hrim Karayei Namaha

[Om Hreem Kah-rah-yei Nahm-ah-hah]

"Om and salutations to She whose seed sound (Hrim) causes the universe to appear or disappear."

653. Om Yoginyei Namaha

[Om Yohg-een-yei Nahm-ah-hah]

"Om and salutations to She who is the power of yoga—union with the divine."

658. Om Iccha Shakti Jnana Shakti Kriya Shakti Swarupinyei Namaha

[Om Ee-chah Shahk-tee Jnah-nah Shahk-tee Kree-yah Shahk-tee Swah-roop-een-yei Nahm-ah-hah]

"Om and salutations to She who is the source of power of the principal shaktis, and all the rest as well."

996. Om Sri Chakra Raja Nilayayei Namaha
[Om Shree Chah-krah Rah-jah Nee-lah-yah-yei
Nahm-ah-hah]
"Om and salutations to She who composes, resides in, and
presides as the Sri Chakra, or Sri Yantra, the great mystic
diagram."

8

Radha
The Power of Divine Love

It is fundamental to Eastern philosophy that Love and Compassion are active forces inherent within humanity. Whether it is the search for the Divine Beloved in meditation or the demonstration of dynamic compassion in humanitarian actions in the world at large, it is our capacity for Love and Compassion that gives evidence of our human divinity. Buddhism emphasizes compassion in all of its branches and teaching. In Buddhism, the final goal of spiritual liberation is itself subordinated to a goal of helping every other sentient being attain its spiritual destiny as its birthright. This is love in action. St. Paul taught that if one does not have love, everything else is nothing, like tinkling brass. Judaism emphasizes charity as a natural outgrowth of love, a form of love in action of which Buddhists highly approve.

Yet given that the idea of love is widely supported, the greater part of humanity lives in misery. Avoiding the political and economic discussions that usually accompany such a statement, I offer to you that the state of happiness wrought by love has nothing to do with economic status. There are beggars who have found so much joy in their devotions that they have chosen to no longer engage in the workaday world. There are humble people living simple lives brimming with loving vitality in the face of every hardship that confronts them. Obviously, it is possible to know love as an internal state that persists under any and all conditions.

Love is the unifying and propagating principle of the cosmos. It shows us our oneness, binds and entwines us inextricably in one another's lives. Manifesting both physically and spiritually, it is the meeting of hearts, of minds, bodies, and souls. It is the highest expression of affinity. It impels us to acts of passion and compassion, and it is also the reward for such acts.

In the Hindu scriptures, there is none who so nearly epitomizes the many faces of love as the eighth avatar of the compassionate Vishnu: Krishna and his power, Radha.

Krishna the Lover

It may be said that Krishna, through his exploits, is as infamous as he is famous. According to the various scriptural accounts in the Puranas and the Mahabharata, Krishna had Radha as a secret lover while still a youth. Later he had two wives, Rukmini and Satyabhama. If this was not enough, he is also said to have had ecstatic union with sixteen thousand *gopis*, or milkmaids. This hardly sounds like the definition of love. Rather, Krishna appears to be a charismatic playboy who uses his charm to gain the affections of many. His behavior seems depraved at worst, opportunistic at best. Such multifarious amorous activities can only cause agony, right? Well, that's not how the story goes. According to the scriptures, the gopis were all completely satisfied. Krishna's lover, Radha, found a way to his side and his wives were not harmed by their husband's widely shared affections, although there was plenty of drama, as we shall see.

The confusing and conflicting stories of these love relationships become clearer when we understand that there are different manifestations of love for each relationship. To begin to unravel the differing kinds of love, we must return to Krishna's previous incarnation as Rama, where he made a promise that could be kept only in the future.

Krishna's Predecessor: Rama

In the myths and legends contained in versions of the *Ramayana* (the life story of Rama and Sita), it is clear that the consciousness of the avatar was not contained in a single body. As the story goes, a divine being appeared before a woman named Kausalya carrying a ball of divine substance that contained the entire consciousness and energy of the coming avatar. The being broke the ball in half, and handed a piece to Kausalya, who consumed it and bore a son, Rama. The remaining portion was broken into more pieces and distributed to Kausalya's sisters. One of the resulting quarters was consumed, and Rama's brother Lakshmana was born. The remaining quarter was again broken, and brothers Bharata and Shatrugna were each born of an eighth. While the entire original ball of divine substance was the energy of the avatar of Vishnu, that energy manifested among several bodies who shared a common consciousness.

Sita, Rama's shakti as Lakshmi incarnate, became Rama's wife. She was discovered one day in the furrow of a field in a neighboring kingdom (in fact, Sita means "one who was found in a furrow"). Thus, the entire avatar was Rama, Lakshmana, Bharata, and Shatrugna, and all their wives or shaktis. Foremost among the shaktis, however, was the incomparable Sita.

As you can see, from the standpoint of the divine ones and their stories, "one body/one consciousness" is not the rule. For them, whatever drama transpired among the brothers and their families, all were in perfect communion at all times.

The part of Rama's story that most pertains to our discussion of love between Krishna and Radha took place as Rama, wandering in exile, searched for Sita, who had been kidnapped. (This episode was foretold by Saraswati at the time of Gayatri's marriage to Brahma.) The same evil ruler who had kidnapped Sita, the demon king Ravana, had also driven many highly advanced sages into the forest, where they now hid. No fewer than sixteen thousand sages, many of them very near to the divine goal of spiritual liberation, were living in small hermitages hidden among the jungle thickets. Rama knew that the sages were hiding there and intentionally sought them out, though he appeared to find them quite by accident.

Meeting Rama, the sages were astonished to discover that they felt an actual physical attraction for him. After a lifetime of asceticism, they were unaccustomed to such urges and did not understand what they were experiencing. Rama explained to them that long-suppressed desires were manifesting because they were very close to liberation. These very last desires must be confronted and somehow completed before they could escape the bondage of karma. Because the Avatar Rama was able to move his consciousness backward and forward in the streams of time, he knew where he had been before, and where he would be in lifetimes to come. Rama told the sages that his spiritual job in his present life forbade him from fulfilling their desires. In this life he was the faithful and loving husband, ruler and spiritual teacher, with perfect behavior in every way. However, he consoled them, in his *next* incarnation, he would fulfill their desires, one of their last prior to liberation.

Fulfilling their last desire just as he had promised, in his incarnation as Krishna, he granted them ecstatic union, then liberated them. Of course, he did not tell them that in order to fulfill those desires they would be born as milkmaids, but from the playful standpoint of Krishna, that would have spoiled everything. There is speculation as to whether Krishna actually made love with the gopis physically, or simply satisfied their desire for union in a metaphysical, spiritual sense. It doesn't matter. He satisfied their hearts' longing while they were still on the physical plane and that satisfaction fulfilled their karma so that they could then be liberated.

This act of love by Krishna is a spiritual love, a transcendental love, even though it played out on the physical plane. The power of that love is Lakshmi, manifesting this time through compassionate lovemaking, in whatever form between Krishna and the gopi-sages. As his shakti, Lakshmi provided Krishna with a never-ending flow of love that easily fulfilled and liberated the sixteen thousand sages, creating rumor, gossip, and a questionable reputation for Krishna in the process. Nonetheless, the power of love provided by Lakshmi through Krishna was unambiguous in its perfect divine purpose. The Sanskrit word for this divine love is *Prema*.

Prema is selfless. In a state of true love, one almost melts away. This is not a negative erasure of the self, but rather a joyous uniting that seems to blur the boundaries between the self and something or someone of great value.

Prema heals. There are many hurts we receive even before we are able to walk and talk, and they continue throughout life. The strength of our species is that we somehow manage to weather them and persevere. Love can heal those hurts, no matter how long ago the wounds were inflected or how deep the scars.

Prema leads to Karma Yoga. Eventually the power of love so unites us with everything and everyone that we are compelled to work toward the fulfillment of others. Such work that seeks to aid others is called the yoga of service, or Karma Yoga. In Buddhism, it takes the form of the Bodhisattva Vow.

Prema is bliss. Whether on the giving or the receiving end, this love embodies complete acceptance. We may find this in another person or in God. While only the perfection of God can completely accept all of our faults and frailties, love with another person can come close, as the joy of sexual union instinctively tells us.

Krishna and Radha in Scriptures

One of the most compelling love relationships in spiritual history comes from the tangled lives of Radha and Krishna. In the various scriptures giving accounts of the love affair between Krishna and his beloved Radha, written over the period of a thousand years, we find several different versions of their relationship. In the *Gita Govinda*, Krishna and Radha are portrayed as a single entity engaged in the difficult task of devising a means of spiritual rescue for humanity during the upcoming (now present-day) spiritual winter known as Kali Yuga, or Age of Strife. In the *Chaura Panchashika*, Radha and Krishna are individual beings who enjoy an illicit love affair. In the *Bhagavata Purana*, the gopis, though satisfied, are disappointed by Krishna's departure from among them. He tells them that his heart belongs to Radha and he must leave. This is also the premise of the *Swadhina Bhartrika*, in which Krishna refers to Radha as "the living Goddess of love's triumph." In the *Vidag Dhamadhava*, Radha threatens suicide because Krishna is leaving her. Although she eventually succeeds in this act, she subsequently returns as the queenly Satyabhama, whom Krishna eventually takes as his second wife.

By the time the *Lalita Madhava* was recorded, Radha's effects were said to extend to the entire universe. The legends surrounding her have come full circle to the place where Radha and Krishna are as one. Radha sees Krishna everywhere, in rocks and trees, streams and birds. In the *Ujjivala Nilamani*, Radha is extolled as even higher than Krishna, because her love is a perfect example of how one should love, with total dedication to the beloved. In fact, it is she who shows that Krishna can be approached by anyone through the vehicle of love.

In the *Brahma Vaivarta*, Krishna declares that he will not grant final liberation to anyone unless they also revere Radha. Devotion to her pleases him even more than devotion to himself. Krishna the avatar is so smitten with Radha that, awed by the quality and completeness of Radha's achievement of love, he mandates that one should propitiate her to achieve his grace. He insists that her love shows the way to liberation and that release will come through devotion to her. Similarly, Radha is completely immersed in Krishna's consciousness. Theirs is a completely mutual love and respect.

It is my view that all of these scriptures present different facets of the diamondlike love between Radha and Krishna, although in the conflicting views they present, a complete understanding of their divinity seems lost. While the pair lived an ostensibly human life, they were really divine and operated from a perspective entirely outside our everyday human view. It's from the perspective of their divinity that we must attempt to look at the events of their lives, the relationship between them, and their effect upon humanity. Therefore, what I present here is a dialogue that synthesizes the various scriptures, written over the period of a thousand years, as they relate to the relationship between Radha and Krishna.

Radha and Krishna Before Embodiment

Lying contentedly under a tree with silken leaves and plump luscious fruit, Vishnu watched the Maxfield Parrish–like sky. Vishnu sighed as vivid blue and iridescent pink clouds drifted by, changing direction and shape at the whim of the etheric universe. It would soon be the time for his next incarnation on Earth before the arrival of Kali Yuga, the spiritual winter of consciousness that would last 432,000 years. Existence then would be troubling, difficult, with short lives, physical and mental diseases, poverty and endless strife revolving around wealth. Yet powered by the shakti of Lakshmi's love, Vishnu's compassion knew no bounds. Somehow, he would find a way to provide a means for humanity to achieve its spiritual birthright. First, he must make his appearance as Krishna and finish some old business, even while he set the stage for events in Kali Yuga.

Closing his eyes momentarily, he reflected on Lakshmi, who had come to him through the swirling mists of the precipitating physical universe those eons and eons ago. Emanating from the bosom of Narayana, that being whose dream from outside all the universes had made them come into existence, Lakshmi had chosen his heart as her abode, placing her power at his disposal. The very thought of her filled him with a warm pulsing current of love and affection for every living thing. Overhead, the bees felt his sentiments and buzzed joyfully from blossom to blossom, feeling the ecstasy of life in every flap of their rapidly moving translucent wings. Brightly colored birds wheeled overhead and dipped their wings in his direction in joyful, unconscious salute.

Pulling himself to an upright position, Vishnu called to Lakshmi with the heartfelt notes of the lover permeating his etheric voice. "O queen of all that exists, kindly show yourself to me in that form in which you first appeared, strolling with such beauty and majesty from that milky ocean. We have important matters to discuss. Besides, that gives me an excuse to behold your beauty in this perfect etheric place. Pray, do not strike me dumb with wonder at the very sight of you, as you did all of us on that day you made your glorious entrance into the cosmos. For although I would just as soon stay forever locked in the embrace of your loving glance, there are conditions coming that command our attention."

A haze of swirling etheric colors danced in front of Vishnu and quickly coalesced into the striking figure of Lakshmi. Ringlets of dark hair exuded exotic perfume. Her beautiful pink sari rested comfortably on a rounded yet delicate form, and her smile lit up the countryside for miles around. "O most compassionate of beings, I am ever here for you. Committed as you are to the welfare of all, I am similarly committed to your welfare. Whether as mother, spouse, lover, or playful companion, I will be whatever you ask." She settled beside him and handed him a piece of ripe fruit she had mischievously hidden behind her.

"However satisfying the taste of this fruit may be, it pales before the taste of you." Vishnu rubbed his cheek with the fruit, then with a playful spirit he grabbed a handful of nearby wildflowers and, pulling off their petals, showered her with a rain of brightly colored flower fragments. For their part, the flowers felt as if their very existence had been sanctified and they expelled perfume to match their blissful state.

Lakshmi laughed and got up quickly. With a darting step she raced to a nearby stream and gathered water in a small pot she carried with her. Returning to her seat in barely a moment, she replied to Vishnu, "Before one can spread flower petals, one must observe the ceremonial oblation." With that, she poured the contents of the pot over Vishnu's head, again laughing the whole time.

Vishnu could not help laughing himself. "Then, since you have performed the oblation, you must now dry me." He grabbed at the hem of her sari and began patting his face. In turn, Lakshmi took a portion of her sari from her shoulder and began to lovingly wipe away the droplets and small puddles of water on Vishnu and his clothes. The two of them then sank into each other's arms and kissed for a very long time.

At length, Lakshmi sat upright and put on a more serious face. "You have asked me to come about a matter of some gravity," she observed.

"Yes," Vishnu replied in a subdued tone. "Kali Yuga, the winter of consciousness, is fast approaching on Earth. Things will not be good there for a long time." He took a bite of the fruit Lakshmi had given him and chewed appreciatively.

"Of course, you will go there," Lakshmi replied matter-of-factly. "And I shall go with you to help."

"The Earth is a beautiful place, but not without hardships," Vishnu observed.

"It is of no consequence. The greater hardship would be for one of us to wait here while the other went there." Lakshmi picked up some flower petals and placed them in a locket she wore around her neck.

"Will you come with me, living in my heart?" Vishnu's eyes smiled.

"You prefer me in a body when you go places." She looked down shyly. "You like people to see me with you."

"Quite true," Vishnu replied.

"Then it is settled," Lakshmi trailed off. "Of course, there is the matter of Saraswati's words at the time of Brahma's wedding to Gayatri. She placed conditions before us that are unalterable."

"I know," replied Vishnu in low tones. "I don't know why I had to open my mouth, it was none of my affair."

"Drama of Narayana, you couldn't help it." Lakshmi flicked a droplet of water at him.

"I agree that there needed to be some way to meet those thousands of sages, but I was not happy to see you kidnapped by that thuggish Ravana."

"Really?" teased Lakshmi. "I thought he was kinda cute."

"Please!" replied Vishnu holding his hand up.

"Well, not that cute." Lakshmi was enjoying herself. "Anyway, it all ended up right. We met those sages, Ravana was defeated, and we gained the throne. Wasn't it a grand time?"

"This will be a bit different." Vishnu was more serious now. "We will be right on the cusp of Kali Yuga. Things will be difficult from the start. Priests will start to charge exorbitant prices for simple ceremonies. Merchants will try to take everything over. Greed will be king and avarice his queen." He shook his head.

"And many saintly souls who are close to liberation will have an easier time of it than ever before, due to the power mantra formulas. 'Nama Eva, Nama Eva' . . ." Lakshmi broke into the Sanskrit axiom declaring the great power of mantra recitation during Kali Yuga. Part of her silently entreated Saraswati and Gayatri to give more power to the practice of mantra in Kali Yuga, since virtue and the ability to focus the mind would be diminished. "And what about those sages? You promised, while living on Earth as Rama, that you would help free them next time."

Vishnu sat silently for a little while. He marveled at the infinite love emanating from Lakshmi. He felt her powerful invocation of Saraswati and Gayatri and knew that in her simple act of love, she had helped millions of souls achieve liberation. Then, in his mind, the drama of his next incarnation on the eve of Kali Yuga began to take shape. He would allow himself to be born to Devaki, who had long yearned for a divine child. Due to ever-watchful King Kamsa's murderous ways, he would have to be removed to another location shortly after birth. "The countryside, that's it. I'll satisfy Saraswati's words by being whisked away to be a cowherd lad." Vishnu smiled.

"And the sages, let them incarnate as milkmaids." Lakshmi's words rang with her loving authority and set into motion the birth of sixteen thousand sages as milkmaids destined to live a rural existence. "Now they'll be close by for you to help them."

Lakshmi grinned engagingly. "I'm even going to be born there myself. . . . So I can help you."

"Good," replied Vishnu, smoothly. "I don't want to ever be that far from you again."

"Think you can handle sixteen thousand at once?" Lakshmi was enjoying this.

"So long as your love empowers me, I can do anything at all."

"Since your nature itself is one of love, then my power merely amplifies what you are already," replied Lakshmi, then changed the subject.

"I think it's my turn to live in multiple bodies. I will copy your example from last time."

"What, exactly, do you mean?" Vishnu was a bit perplexed.

"Well, last time you incarnated in Lakshmana, Bharata, and Shatrugna as well as Rama," she stated matter-of-factly.

"Yes, that's true." Vishnu still did not see where this was leading.

"This time I will incarnate in several bodies, just as you did!" Lakshmi clapped her hands in delight. "I will come while you are young, as your Divine Beloved Radha—illicit, yet satisfying all at once. You will hunger for me like no other. Then I will send part of me to be your rightful queen Rukmini—divine, lovely, powerful, and radiant. That part of me will not want to let you out of my sight lest you find me as Radha."

"You are ever my beloved no matter what form you take. You know that we will be separated when I must leave to fight in the war between the Yadhavas and the Pandavas. You will be just as inconsolable as I was when Ravana kidnapped you." Vishnu adeptly changed the subject.

"When you are still young and leave me as Radha, I will take my own life and quickly be reborn. Later, as a grown man, you will take me as your second wife, Satyabhama. As her, I will save your life when the time comes. I love to throw a little Durga in here and there for emphasis." Lakshmi gazed into the tableau of the future and set forces into motion that would make events take the course she had just uttered.

"My love, I have not decided yet how best to rid the world of the evil King Kamsa." Vishnu bit his lip in concentration.

"Oh, that's easy. When you leave for the countryside, I'll come as Durga, the Divine Protectress. When Kamsa comes to investigate, I'll just dispatch him on the spot. A jolt from my big toe should take care of him." Lakshmi instantly carved out the future with short phrases.

At the thought of Lakshmi killing Kamsa, that big, hairy, and smug oaf of a ruler, with her big toe Vishnu laughed out loud. "Oh, do it when people are around!" he urged. "Somebody has to see it!"

"Sage Narada will see it. In fact, when we're done I'm going to go tell him everything we're going to do. Knowing him, he won't be able to resist needling Kamsa for years before the actual event, foretelling of his destruction and death." Lakshmi had great affection for the wandering sage Narada, and cherished his intricate meddling that always produced such breathtaking results in the affairs of celestials and mortals alike. He quickened the evolutionary power of the divine wherever he went.

"So, what will you do when Kali Yuga actually begins?" Lakshmi lovingly inquired of Vishnu about his subsequent incarnation even before the next had begun.

"Oh, I don't know. But I'll find a way to get rid of a lot of those Brahmin priests, I can tell you that. The good ones are like divine nectar, but the majority are just greedy and power hungry. I'll just have to do some kind of housecleaning." Vishnu knew he would enjoy that incarnation. He was already outlining his work when he would come as the Buddha.

"And after that?" Lakshmi pressed on.

"By that time humanity should be about ready to take care of themselves. Then I can dally here endlessly with you." His love-filled eyes held hers.

"I cherish that coming moment, my love. But you will need to go there during Kali Yuga, or send some help from time to time."

"I will send my friend Uddhava. He is completely devoted to me and will do what I ask."

"I'll always be there to help." Lakshmi returned Vishnu's gaze with her own radiant love. "Should I go with Uddhava?" she teased.

Vishnu was momentarily startled. "Why would you even suggest such a thing!"

Laughing because she had tripped him up, if only for a moment, Lakshmi clarified things. "I will send one of my very own devoted handmaids, with a part of my essence, to be spouse to your dependable and devoted Uddhava. Just as you always have me, he shall always have her."

"Now that the details are settled, let's rehearse. I will be Krishna and you will be Radha. First, let's make love for about a hundred years. Then we can rest on each other's lap for another hundred. After that . . ." And so Vishnu choreographed the next act in a divine love story that would go on for thousands of years to come. Lakshmi, as the power of his love, would make changes in his scenario as they were needed.

Mantras for Love

As portrayed in the various scriptures written about them, Radha (an emanation of Lakshmi) and Krishna enjoy a quintessential personal love relationship. For her part, Radha-Lakshmi knows she is empowering Krishna-Vishnu in all of his actions. Since he also knows this, he treats her with the complete respect commensurate with her status as his complement. We all have the potential to create the same kind of relationship here on Earth. When we realize that the feminine shakti in any personal relationship has a supercharging effect upon all of our activities, we will then treat the person who holds that shakti with great respect. If the objective in our personal relationship is to love each other as equals while each recognizes the other person's special contributions, we are on the right track to experience a great personal love.

For Building a Soaring Conjugal Love on the Earth Plane

1. Om Radha Krishnaya Namaha
[Om Rahd-hah Krish-nah-yah Nahm-ah-hah]
"Om and salutations to that single being of Love, manifesting as the lovers Radha and Krishna."

To expect immediate transformation of an abusive relationship into a healthy one is not a realistic expectation for this or any other mantra. But this mantra can be used by either partner of a marriage for the gradual but sure improvement of the overall relationship. Care and intimacy can be greatly enhanced. This mantra also works powerfully in relationships where there is genuine commitment between the two people.

In the story above, Vishnu adores Lakshmi and showers love upon her. Lakshmi adores Vishnu and empowers both his heart's love and the divine abilities that will enable him to help others. Similarly, we can adore one another, shower love upon one another, and help one another accomplish those things that are dear to us.

For Bringing the Highest Possible Expression of Love into Your Life

2. Om Parama Prema Rupaya Namaha
[Om Pah-rah-mah Prei-mah Roo-pah-yah Nahm-ah-hah]
"Om and salutations to the supreme divine love, coming in a recognizable form."

The love invoked by this mantra may or may not be sexual in character. I knew a woman many years ago who used this mantra. She attracted a spiritual teacher, or guru, with whom she had sex on several occasions. Even after they physically parted and she left to marry and have children, she always felt his love and protection with her. His loving presence was a constant inspiration and source of guidance for her, even many years later.

This does not mean that one should necessarily approve of or condone such sexual activities. The importance of this incident is the love that came from it, a love that lasted a long time even after the sexual part was over. We may also come into a relationship where the sexual part, for one reason or another, comes to an end. But it need not be the end of our love.

This mantra may also bring an ecstatic vision of the divine beloved.

For Becoming the Highest Form of Love You Can Be

3. Aham Prema
[Ah-hum Prei-mah]
"I am Divine Love."

With this simple mantra, you affirm your own essential nature as one of Divine Love. The vibration of this mantra begins the process of transforming your entire body, being, nature, and spirit into an emanation, your own particular emanation, of Divine Love. I know a man who had meditated for many, many years before he started saying this mantra. After chanting it for just a few weeks, he told me that he felt as if he were being "filled" with love. He felt increasing love for his wife and family. He noticed that his desire in everyday situations was to become the transforming force of love. He felt love becoming a force in his business activities as well as his personal life. He wondered out loud where it was going to lead, even as his smile told us both he already knew the answer.

There are others who have used this mantra and reported back to me weeks and months later that they felt some inner transformation was happening that defied description. They all agreed that, whatever it was, they liked it a lot.

9

Kuan Yin
The Power of Divine Compassion

If personal love fulfills, heals, and transforms, then compassion is a state of elevation beyond personal love. If one is satisfied in every way, personal love has achieved all of its desires. Then, for some, the focus of attention may move from oneself to others, and we may start to ask questions: What about the other people I know, do they have love, this blossoming of the heart? Should not everyone experience this state?

Following in the footsteps of these questions may come the life-altering question: If other people do not have love or proper life conditions, is there something I can do to help? The moment this question appears in the mind, everything changes.

The power of a personal love begins an alchemical transformation into the power of compassion. It grows, warms, and extends itself to all sentient beings, regardless of their location, species, or level of development. It becomes, in a word, universal. It contains sympathy, but is so much more. It contains empathy, but on a scale outside everyday considerations. It contains knowledge, but of a transcendent quality that knows not only the destination but also the right road to travel. It adapts itself to any circumstance the way water seeks always to flow into any crevice until it fills and reaches every level. Finally, compassion is a dynamic quality. Sensation and sentiment are not enough, one must also act, give aid.

The roots of this exceptionally noble power are found in the myth of Avalokiteshwara, who is traditionally portrayed as the epitome of compassion.

Avalokiteshwara the Compassionate

Somewhere in the vast reaches of one of the infinite number of space-time continua, a being named Avalokiteshwara labored toward the zenith of its spiritual potential as a conscious entity. Physicality had been transcended. Intellect had been expanded. Intuition had blossomed into concrete knowledge of higher worlds and the means to attain them. Powers of the mind had evolved, transcending the human idea of a solitary finite existence. What we call emotion was fired in the crucible of experience until it became a distillation of pure love. Unity was understood as a thread that bound together all the realms of all continua and all the conscious species.

One day, Avalokiteshwara reached a place within itself that is impossible to understand in the way that this being experienced it. By way of analogy, we could say that Avalokiteshwara, through all the travails of conscious striving, realizations, spiritual evolution, and attainment, finally reached a place that was like climbing a very high mountain. Upon reaching the summit, a high stone wall was encountered. By piling up convenient boulders and loose rocks, Avalokiteshwara finally scaled the top of the fence and looked over to the other side. The view that presented itself to Avalokiteshwara's understanding was utterly confounding and attractive at the same time. It was obvious that Avalokiteshwara should jump into that which lay on the other side of the wall. It represented the end of all striving. It was the goal, liberation, the final step for all of Avalokiteshwara's existence.

Just as the being was about to leap into that place, it heard a sound emanating from behind it, near the foot of the mountain. Avalokiteshwara hesitated for a moment, and turned around. The sound came again like a low, forceful moan of great sorrow and despair. In an instant Avalokiteshwara understood the sound's meaning. The collective unconscious of sentient beings everywhere realized that it was about to lose the presence of this great being from among its number. By jumping over the fence, Avalokiteshwara would be gone forever from the field of activity occupied by other sentient beings at whatever their level of attainment. The great elevated consciousness and force for good would return no more.

As Avalokiteshwara heard and understood the meaning of the moan, the element of dynamic compassion that was the very nature of this being asserted itself, and a decision was made. There would be no jump over the fence. Climbing down from the pile of boulders, Avalokiteshwara became the Bodhisattva of Compassion (a Bodhisattva is an individual who has become the essence of wisdom and delays his or her, or, as in the case of Avalokiteshwara, *its* final stage of enlightenment or release from the wheel of existence as an individual being in order to serve, to aid the progress of the multitudes who come behind). From this initial compassionate act comes what has since become known as the Bodhisattva Vow. Although there are different versions with minor variations, its essence is:

"I postpone final beatification, the final stage of complete enlightenment, the last step of evolution for any conscious being, and dedicate my existence to the benefit and progress of conscious, sentient beings everywhere. I will work for their opportunity to attain what I have attained. One day, all sentient beings will stand where I now stand. Then, we will all jump over this last wall together."

Anyone who consistently practices any Buddhist technique from any lineage, from any country, will one day be presented with an opportunity to take the Bodhisattva Vow. It is no small thing. If you feel inspired to take the vow, it means that within you are the same sentiments that gripped Avalokiteshwara at the top of the mountain: a profound caring for your fellows that would prevent you from accepting final personal release until all may be released. Taking the vow would mean that you are now committed to the great task of helping others attain enlightenment. You would join what some have called The Work in your own way.

That we are each imperfect in our attainments does not matter. That we may have humble ways and means to contribute to The Work also does not matter. It is the depth of our sincerity and commitment that is important. Knowledge can be ephemeral, appearing and disappearing like the sun on cloud-strewn days. Love, similarly, can seem transient, as loved ones are born and die, as relationships form and fade. Siddhis (divine abilities) may come and go according to karma, astrology, and divine intervention. But divine love and wisdom that have been transformed into compassion can remain under any and all conditions. And work founded in dynamic compassion always receives the blessings of the celestials, the angels, the saints, the true gurus, the masters, and the army of servants of God who often travel in disguise.

The Mantra

The Buddha Amitabha is said to be a conscious force in the universe that assumes a given form simply so that it may thus be contemplated. The Buddhist legend, contained in scriptures from

India such as the *Sad Dharma Pundarika Sutra*, is that Avalokiteshwara is one such emanation of Amitabha, a Bodhisattva conjured
by Amitabha that we might contemplate that state of existence.
In this legend, Avalokiteshwara, holding a lotus blossom, springs
from a ray coming from the right eye of Amitabha and immediately begins to chant the great Mani mantra.

The Great Mani Mantra

1. Om Mani Padme Hum
[Om Mah-nee Pahd-may Hoom]
"Om. The Jewel of Consciousness has reached the Heart's
Lotus."

In Eastern spiritual circles, there is a saying that when mind
and heart are united, anything is possible. This mantra is extraordinarily powerful in linking the capacities of the mind with the
divinity in the heart. It is the human capacity born of mind linking with heart that accounts for the transforming power of compassion. It is a state from which, thankfully, there is no turning back.

Repeated more than any other mantra in the world, millions of
devoted Buddhists chant this mantra every day, sometimes for
hours at a time. Through this practice, they are actively working
not only for their own spiritual advancement but for yours and
mine as well. For this mantra has the effect of elevating incremen-
tally the mental/emotional environment around the planet each
and every time it is chanted.

It is heartbreaking that the Chinese incursion into Tibet has
driven thousands of monks from the monasteries and imprisoned
or killed millions of others. The karma incurred from such acts
must be dreadful indeed. But many of the exiled Tibetans have
come to the West as teachers and inspired hundreds of thousands

of us to chant these powerful formulas that, with other Sanskrit mantras, will eventually change the vibration of the planet itself. Even from this brutal tragedy, some good has come.

Kuan Yin

Returning to the story of Avalokiteshwara, the *Sad Dharma Pundarika Sutra* recounts 337 different human incarnations of this being, most of which were male and manifested in Tibet. But in China this being is considered feminine. In China, a Buddhist scholar named Kumar Rajiva, in his translation of the Lotus Sutra in A.D. 406, first officially designated an incarnation of Avalokiteshwara, Kuan Yin, as female. In this telling, seven of the 33 human incarnations of Avalokiteshwara are feminine, with Kuan Yin being the most widely recognized. By the ninth century, temples and shrines to Kuan Yin had been built throughout China, all depicting her in feminine form.

Kuan Yin is often called "She who hears the cries of the world," which in part certainly refers to the legend of Avalokiteshwara, who put off a final evolutionary step in the story just told. But in the fabric of daily life in China, Kuan Yin is much more down to earth in helping with everyday matters, not just in reaching the spiritual heights. Here is a Chinese folktale explaining the genesis of Avalokiteshwara as Kuan Yin.*

Many centuries ago, an unnamed governor living in a remote province had a daughter of whom he was quite fond. As a Taoist conservative, however, he kept his daughter under restraint in the household and forbade her travel outside the confines of his offices on the gubernatorial grounds.

---

*A longer version of this story appears in *Bodhisattva of Compassion: The Mystical Tradition of Kuan Yin*, by John Blofeld (Boston: Shambhala Publications, 1988).

Sitting near her upstairs apartment window, the daughter viewed the world over the wall surrounding the grounds and contemplated what lay beyond the gates. She was particularly intrigued by the towers of a monastery she saw off in the distance. Inspired by the outward beauty of the place, she wondered what grand mystic ceremonies and observances must take place in the inner worship chambers. Whenever she mentioned these thoughts to her attendants or her father's staff, they would quickly change the subject, ignoring her comments altogether.

At length she decided to go to the monastery to investigate it for herself. Disguising herself as a servant girl, she left the grounds by a seldom-used gate and traveled the mile or so to the gleaming temple gates. Not at all fooled by her slight disguise, the gateman let her inside, thinking that this rich young woman might have valuable gifts for the temple. She was directed toward the main shrine without delay. There the young woman was delighted at the sight of the statues of Three Pure Ones, a trinity of Taoist deities, and smiled at the charming melodies that echoed through the hall. Thinking she was possessed of great good fortune to be in the company of saints, she joyously roamed the grounds with its gardens, small out-of-the-way shines, and dimly lit corridors. She had no idea that the saints there were few. Instead, most of the monks practiced swordplay by day and bedroom games by night. Soon she was surrounded by a group of monks and forced into a room off one of the many small corridors honeycombing the grounds. Her screams were drowned out by the sounds of ceremonies coming from a nearby shrine.

At her father's home there was now concern over the whereabouts of the missing girl. The governor suspected she might have left the grounds and sent out search parties to inquire. Word soon came back that a young woman had, indeed, visited the temple earlier in the day, but she was not there now.

The governor was not convinced. He had his own theory about his daughter meeting with a lover at the temple, for the lasciviousness of the monks was well known. With hard purpose he decided to rid the area of the masquerading holy men as well as his wayward daughter. Lining up archers at every entrance and giving instructions that anyone leaving should be shot, he ordered the temple set on fire. The wooden structures were soon gobbled by the spreading flames.

Early the next morning the governor strolled in his private gardens trying to ignore the guilt he felt for killing his own daughter. Suddenly, the form of a dead child appeared in a hazy glow and it spoke to him.

"O Father, you had no pity on a young girl who did not escape being violated. Even so, I cannot help having pity on you. No more children shall be born to you, thus I will bring you comfort in my present state. I tell you now that heaven was compassionate toward my undeserved suffering. While the monastery burned, I was rescued and taken above the clouds to the domain of the celestial ones. There, according to the Law of Compensation invoked to counter my undeserved fate, I was elevated to the position of goddess. I will now comfort those who are afflicted and save those in jeopardy, as I was. Hereafter, I shall become known as Kuan Shi Yin, She who hears the cries of the world."

People pray to Kuan Yin for all kinds of things using the mantra given below. Businesspeople propitiate her to prosper. Chinese families pray for her help in ironing out complicated, duty-oriented obligations that are more convoluted than any American soap opera. Thus, even though the Lotus Sutra proclaims that she travels the world to help beings to enlightenment, she often will offer grace in the most seemingly insignificant problems, if it relieves the suffering of those involved.

An engaging story, told by John Blofeld in *Bodhisattva of Compas-*

sion: The Mystical Tradition of Kuan Yin, centers around a Chinese man educated in British Catholic schools who subsequently returned to China and was almost immediately engulfed in the effects of the Japanese invasion during World War II. Sent to work miles off the main road in the remote province of Kweichow, he took a wrong turn while his party was trudging through endless low mountain passes. He soon realized he was lost, but since he could see fresh piles of mule dung on the path he was following, he assumed his party must be just ahead.

As he slowly ascended into deepening mists and increasing cold, an icy wind cut through his clothing and the man realized he was in trouble. Still, he was not sure he should retrace his steps. He heard faint animal sounds, and the cold grew more intense. Finally, he dropped to his knees and prayed to St. Bernadette, begging her to lead him to safety.

In his mind, he thought of the saint as a sweet child, full of grace and mercy. As he prayed, he suddenly saw her standing on a flat rock, the thin blue pajamas she was wearing scarcely fluttering in the increasing howl of wind and snow. She was smiling and around her a glow of light shimmered in the deepening evening. Then he noticed something odd. Bernadette was Chinese, with high-swept hair and jewels about her throat. After just a moment, she spoke to him, telling him that she would lead him to a place of safety for the night. Following her for less than a quarter of a mile, they arrived at a small, protected cave where she told him he would be safe. The floor of the cave was soft with layers of silky soft dirt, upon which he immediately fell asleep.

When he awoke the next morning, the day was clear and bright. Looking down, he observed that the floor of the cave was pitted, rocky, sharp, and almost dangerous. Yet he had slept upon it in comfort. As he emerged from the cave and went to wash in a nearby stream, a mule train passed by from which he received both food and directions back down to the place where he had strayed from the proper path.

A few years after this event, the man was traveling in another province when a cloudburst sent him running for the shelter of a seldom-used local temple. There he came upon a faded fresco of Kuan Yin, depicted as a simple young woman, dressed in the same blue silk pajamas he had seen in his vision on the mountain path years ago. The image in the painting was identical in every way to the vision of she who had saved him, except for the jewels around the neck, which were missing from the fresco. The man realized that it was she, Kuan Yin, and not St. Bernadette, who had appeared to him in his hour of need, full of compassion and giving real-world aid.

Kuan Yin Mantra

I have chanted the Kuan Yin mantra and performed Kuan Yin ceremonies since 1985, and the feeling it generates is unique among the mantras I use. It produces a feeling of calm within minutes. Among mantras used in the East, this one has traditionally been used primarily in China and Japan, only becoming popular in the English-speaking world through John Blofeld in the 1970s. It is unique in that it is used as an all-purpose mantra, chanted for any difficulty, problem, or desire.

Kuan Yin Mantra

1. **Namo Kuan Shi Yin Pu Sa**
[Nah-moh Kwahn Shee Yin Poo Sah]
"Salutations to the most compassionate and merciful Bodhisattva Kuan Yin."

Each time I perform one of the many Sanskrit ceremonies I conduct for people, the experience is unique. However, a Kuan Yin water ceremony that I performed in early 2000 stands out clearly in memory. In front of those who attended the ceremony, I spread out a plastic cloth and put in place a number of copper plates, pots, spoons, cups, and other ceremonial paraphernalia, with each item having a specific purpose. The centerpiece of the ceremony is the pouring of ceremonial oblations (water or milk, for example) over the murti, a religious icon or statue that symbolically represents the purpose of the ceremony we are performing. I came across this particular Kuan Yin murti when Margalo and I attended a gem show in Santa Monica. There in one of the display booths was a beautiful foot-high, violet-colored, translucent ceramic statue of Kuan Yin. I admired the statue greatly, so Margalo immediately bought it from the Chinese vendor and gave it to me, saying, "Happy Father's Day!"

As I set up for the ceremony, a process I have gone through literally thousands of times, I found that I could not contain my joy. I was feeling something so wonderful that I was glad to be able to share it with others. Then, as I sat down, closed my eyes, and intoned the opening mantras, I felt something come over my head. It was really an odd feeling. It was almost as if I were suddenly wearing a stiff shawl or was crammed into some shallow rock shelf.

Opening my eyes, my glance fell to the plate at my side on which sat the beautiful image of Kuan Yin. Her carved pose in the statue suggested someone who had a stiff shawl over her head or was sitting on a shallow rock shelf. My feeling was in exact correspondence with her pose. For a second, I was speechless, then I resumed the ceremony. For the rest of the service, I felt that I was somehow in union with the statue of Kuan Yin. I concentrated intensely to do the best job I possibly could. If I was somehow connected with the image of Kuan Yin, then I wanted everything coming out of my mouth to be as perfect as possible for the benefit of those who were assembled. When the ceremony was over, the feeling subsided. Although a number of people commented on the beauty and the power of the ceremony, such statements are not uncommon. But for me, the ceremony was anything but commonplace. In no other has there ever been anything like that feeling, before or since.

Use the Kuan Yin mantra to invoke her assistance for any difficulty whatsoever. Both in mainland China and on Taiwan, the faithful have been calling on her for help and receiving her assistance. But she has promised to respond to anyone in difficulty, anywhere in the world.

10

Tara
The Power of the Divine Mother

In 1975, I was summoned from Washington, D.C., to Los Angeles to be a priest for a new local chapter of a fledgling organization called Sanatana Vishwa Dharma. The chapter lasted all of five months. When it became clear, after just a few weeks, that the Los Angeles branch would close, I salved my disappointment by visiting the Los Angeles County Museum of Art, where an exhibit of Tibetan art was in progress.

Although I had learned a substantial amount of history and principles pertaining to Vedic Hinduism, I knew nothing at all about Tibetan Buddhism. I didn't know the gods and goddesses, the history, or anything else about this wondrous mountain world. But I was interested, nonetheless, in the icons and *thankas* (paintings on cloth) so unique to Tibet.

As I wandered through the halls, visiting first one set of figures, then another, a thanka hanging on a wall on the other side of the hall attracted my attention. Why that one? I moved to follow the energy of the painting that was obviously calling to me. When I arrived, I saw a feminine figure sitting in the midst of a complicated *mandala* (diagram). She was green, radiant, and had a look on her face that defied description even as it calmed me in some inexplicable way. Within seconds I was drawn into a meditative state in which I just stared at her form and face while I stood there for a long time. After somewhere between twenty and forty minutes, a woman from the organization, who had accompanied me to the museum, tapped me on the shoulder. She looked at me in the oddest way and wondered out loud how long I had been there. I said I didn't know, but that I felt I was in tune with something or someone that was completely concerned for my welfare.

With the closing of the local chapter, those of us who lived there had to find new quarters. Since I had no job other than temple priest, I was completely without funds. Within three days of my museum trip, I was invited back to Washington, D.C., to serve as temple priest there. Within another ten days, I was offered a part-time teaching job at George Washington University. I felt that the grace and compassion of the universe responded and lifted me from that place. One could say that it was the Grace of the Mother, and I would not argue.

Avalokiteshwara, Kuan Yin, and Tara

In Tibet, the story of Avalokiteshwara, the Bodhisattva of Compassion, is very well known and propitiated in his masculine form, Chenresig. In China and Japan, the feminine form of Kuan Yin is best known. But in all three countries and in both masculine and feminine forms, the power of compassion is invoked using the Great Mani Mantra, "Om Mani Padme Hum."

There is another figure closely related to both Kuan Yin and Avalokiteshwara (or Chenresig), a towering figure whose fame spreads even beyond the East. This is Tara, Mother of the World. Tara's eminence is of long standing in Tibet and certain provinces of Mongolia, but her fame elsewhere is both ancient and quite recent, however puzzling that might sound at first.

Many of the attributes of Tara and Kuan Yin are strikingly similar. Both are appealed to for almost any difficulty or problem. Assessments of their powers seem to range between the fantastic and near absolute. That the aspect of compassion is the very foundation of their nature is near proof of the adage that compassionate love conquers all. In their iconography are clues to their differences, although as we shall shortly see, early iconography provides clues that there may be a common root between the two goddesses as well.

The representations of Kuan Yin show her with a lotus, with a child, with a great fish, pouring forth the waters of blessing from a small vial, among other traditional poses. Sometimes she is standing and sometimes seated in an almost heroic pose that is androgynous or even masculine in appearance.

Tara almost always is shown sitting in a very specific posture, one that resembles a loose yogic pose. While she, too, often holds flowers, her manner of displaying these is distinct from poses shown in Kuan Yin iconography. Tara is master of mudra, or divine gesture. In this spiritual art of movement, different hand poses project different kinds of energy. While Kuan Yin is depicted always with the same one or two mudras, Tara is shown with a far greater variety, suggesting that her powers, too, are of a far greater variety.

John Blofeld hypothesizes that at one time Kuan Yin and Tara may have been the same entity. Via a route that we may not be able to accurately trace, he postulates that Kuan Yin came to be known in China while the feminine depiction of a great savioress evolved as Tara in Tibet. Blofield wrote in *Kuan Yin: Bodhisattva of Compassion*: "Visiting Japan . . . I chanced upon three early paintings of Kuan Yin, or Kwannon-Sama as she is known in that country. For several reasons there could be no doubt that the figure depicted was Kuan Yin, but her posture and the mudras formed by her fingers were those of Tara! Moreover, in the British

Museum there is a painting in which the central figure is clearly that of Kuan Yin, for she is accompanied by her Chinese disciples Shan Ts'ai and Lung Nu, but again her posture is Tara's! Clearly these painting belonged to an era when the forms of Tara and Kuan Yin began to merge. . . . To scholars and art lovers, the details of iconography are of great significance."*

Tara, the Power of the Universal Mother

It would not be a mistake to refer to Tara as the Universal Mother because, as mentioned briefly above, her fame is not restricted to Tibet or Buddhist teachings. Traces of her can be found nearly the world over.

The Druids of Old Britain also called their mother goddess Tara, and ancient Finnish legends speak of the goddess Tar. A tribe in the South American jungles calls their goddess Tara Humara. References to her are so numerous and widespread that some linguists have wondered if the Latin word *terra*, for earth, somehow had its roots in the Sanskrit word *tara*, meaning star. Legends told by the American Cheyenne Indians speak of a "star woman" who fell to Earth from the Heavens, out of whose body grew all essential food.

To Tibetans she is known simply as The Mother, The Savioress, and The Protectress. There are numerous accounts of her assisting the Tibetan refugees who fled the Chinese occupation of their homeland. Many stories contain the following type of scenario:

The fleeing Tibetans come to a place where their path splits in two, one through a valley, the other over a high pass. Although

---

* John Blofeld, *Bodhisattva of Compassion: The Mystical Tradition of KuanYin* (Boston: Shambhala Publications, 1978), pages 41–42.

the divergent paths rejoin farther on, one must be chosen to follow now. The refugees choose the path indicated by Tara in one of the party's dream, only later to hear of a Chinese patrol that they narrowly missed by following Tara's instructions. Another typical Tara story is that of a monk who, while in deep meditation, received a message from Tara insisting that a planned trip be delayed. The monk is warned that there will be disaster if the party leaves as planned. So the departure was set back a week. Two days later, a huge snowstorm moved in. If they had left on their original schedule, the party would have been trapped, stranded, and possibly died.

Tara's Various Aspects

Although there are a total of twenty-one Taras found in Tibetan lore, she is primarily worshiped today in two forms: the Green Tara and the White Tara. Her most famous representation is as Green Tara, the dynamic aspect of compassion propitiated to overcome difficulties of all kinds. Called The Mother of the Buddhas—past, present, and future—Tara is found everywhere, irrespective of sect, creed, or particular Buddhist practice. She sits on the private altar of monks throughout the world, regardless of the order to which they belong.

In mental disciplines for which the Tibetans are renowned, Tara is often described as a dynamically powerful archetype for our own inner wisdom. Here, Tara is an instrument for transformation of consciousness, another kind of journey to spiritual freedom.

Tara protects those who call to her with her mantras, but she also knows very well how to take care of herself. A recent Nepalese newspaper carried the story of a citizen of Great Britain who paid 400,000 Nepalese rupees (about $4,000) for a magnificent image of holy Tara measuring slightly more than a foot in height.

The man attempted to smuggle the image illegally out of the country by placing it inside a carry-on bag that was not opened by airport inspection. But as the man proceeded toward his gate, his bag grew heavier and heavier until he was forced to drop it and was unable to lift it again. This alerted the Nepalese officials who opened the bag to inspect it. Finding Tara's statue inside, they immediately confiscated it.

The White Tara is also often referred to as the Mother of the Buddha, particularly as the motherly aspect of compassion. Her distinguishing characteristic is vigilance, a vigilance that reaches everywhere. She sees through seven different eyes—the usual two and the mystic third eye between the brows, as well as an eye on the palm of each hand, and one on the sole of each foot. Artistic renderings of her show these eyes as well as the lotus of compassion that she holds. Most thankas show Tara displaying the divine mudra (hand gesture) signifying the three jewels of Buddhism: the Buddha (a state of consciousness, rather than any one individual), Dharma (divine law), and *Sangha* (spiritual fellowship). White Tara is also said to be able to grant long life. The following is a list of the twenty-one qualities or aspects of Tara according to their color manifestations.

White Tara
   Destroys poison
   Makes one invincible
   Emanates various rays of light
   Gives deep peace
   Bestows divine creativity
   Long life

Pale Pink Tara
   Savioress of the scented forest
   Destroyer of opposing forces

Conqueror of the worldly realms
Swiftest of heroines
She who blesses mountain-dwelling mendicants

Light Brown Tara
She who ensures victory
Giver of supreme virtue
She who is auspiciousness itself

Dark Brown Tara
Giver of intelligence
She who subdues evil spirits
She who conquers those who stand in the way of spiritual advancement

Dark Tan Tara
Blazing light
Provider of wealth

Jet Black Tara
Wrathful protectress against hidden enemies
She who is invincible in relieving suffering

Green Tara
Mother of the Buddhas and incomparable savioress

The roots of Tara's veneration are not entirely clear. Because she predates the advent of writing, we are dependent upon the accuracy of an oral tradition. Although scholars traditionally do not accept stories handed down orally with as much confidence as they do written records, often these tales are all we have to go on.

Documented research has concluded that Tara had already

been firmly established by A.D. 630, when Avalokiteshwara was said to have disguised himself as King Songsten Gampo. Covering ten of his heads so that only one appeared, his two wives were said to be emanations of Tara. His Chinese wife, Wen Cheng Kung Chu, was said by Kunga Dorje in the Buddhist text *Red Annals* to be an emanation of White Tara, while his Nepalese wife, Tr'itsun, was an emanation of Green Tara. Before her appearance in Nepal and Tibet, Wen Cheng Kung Chu is reported to have exhibited signs of compassion for the common people and later would be declared an emanation of Tara. Still later, there are historical reports of a Chinese pilgrim, Hsuan Tsang, who went into India between 633 and 645 and reported that he found temples dedicated to one who he concluded was none other than their very own Chinese Tara. This anecdote agrees with history as the Tibetans teach it.

Veneration of Tara persisted in Tibet through a succession of righteous kings, until Langdharma was assassinated in 836 and the new king decreed that her "secret charms were to be translated no longer." This stringent policy was persistently enforced through petty rulers until 1042. As a result, we have no definitive proof that Tara was known beyond the walls of the monastery until her popularization through Sage Atisha.

Mystical Tara Appears

Around 1040, Atisha, a young boy born to aristocratic parents, had a vision of Tara. She appeared to him again and again in dreams and meditations in which she exhorted the lad to give up his abundant material heritage and travel to another country, where he would find new spiritual teachings. Tara told Atisha that although he would have a shorter life by making this trip, he would gain great merit by helping many beings.

Thus encouraged by Tara, Atisha traveled and met the great teacher Dharmakirti (whose name means "famous law"), and mastered many levels of Buddhist instruction and practice. He subsequently traveled on alone to Tibet, where he established the teachings pertaining to Tara that we know today. Of the 117 sacred texts Atisha wrote, only 4 were devoted to Tara. And of the 67 he translated from the original Sanskrit into Tibetan, only 6 dealt with Tara. The reason for this apparent neglect was political. The ruling council in Tibet forbade Atisha to teach certain methods of practice and invocation that he learned from another teacher, Hayagriva (the same sage who taught the mysteries of Lalita to Agastya). Specifically, Atisha was forbidden to reveal the Tantra of Tara the Yogini, source for all rituals and wellspring of secret teachings, to anyone. It is interesting that Hayagriva gave the same warning about release of the power of the Great Feminine to Atisha that he gave to Agastya.

From the time of the arrival of Atisha, the branches of Tibetan Buddhism that we recognize today took hold and have flourished ever since. Each branch can trace its connection to Tara.

Ningma—This lineage can trace scriptures and worship by its leaders back to the earliest times and practices. It is the oldest sect, often called the ancient sect. The three sects that follow grew out of the Buddhist renaissance sparked by Atisha.

Gelupta—Members of this branch adhere to the teachings of Atisha and consider themselves pure in their approach.

Sakya—Tara, the patron saint of this theology, is also considered to have an emanation called Kurukulla, the Mistress of Potent Subjugation, whose mantra is given in the *Hvega Tantra*.

Kagyu—Gampopa, the progenitor of this lineage, was a direct disciple of Atisha. Through revelation of Tara, the Karmapas were empowered and have presided over this branch of Tibetan Buddhism to the present day.

Hindu Roots, Buddhist Roots

The oral tradition's contribution to the lore of Tara holds some surprises. In some stories, Tara is described as an ogress, in others as "the morning star." As an ogress, she was said to possess an insatiable lust, and sexually importuned a resistant leader of the Monkey Clan again and again. Frustrated, she finally threatened to eat a thousand monkeys every day. The leader of the monkeys at last complied and satisfied her carnal desires. It turned out to be a blessing.

As a result of this mating between Tara and the leader of the Monkey Clan, their offspring became more intelligent as well as compassionate. Because of their increased intellectual abilities, subsequent leaders and kings were able to "receive" knowledge of the methods and techniques of certain crafts from a divine source. Over several generations, using these new skills, villages were created that eventually would become Tibetan society.

In this story, told in the *Red Annals*, composed in 1346, the Monkey leader is the first disciple of Avalokiteshwara. To this day, many older Tibetans believe that humanity descended from this mating of the ancient ogress and the monkey.

As I encountered this tale of Tara, my mind turned to the *Ramayana*, the life story and exploits of the Avatar Rama. In this book, the foremost servant of Rama is Hanuman, a monkey, in a society that, according to the oral tradition, existed some seven thousand years ago.

The Tibetan myths say that in an earlier time Tara had helped two monkey chieftains, Sugriva and Angada. Now, Sugriva is clearly named in the *Ramayana* as one of its supporting characters. Here was a link between that ancient time of Rama and the stories surrounding Tara in modern Tibet. In the *Ramayana*, Sugriva was a monkey king who was having a difficult time ruling until Rama appeared and helped him out. Is there some correlation between Tara and Rama?

A Fallen Star?

Among the most advanced Hindu mystical teachers, there is no disagreement that the Avatar Rama, as an avatar of Vishnu, was not from here. That is to say that, although he had a human-appearing body, he was not human in the sense that we are. The same is most emphatically true of Krishna. Many Indian mystics speculate that Sage Hayagriva was also not human, that he came from elsewhere and looked quite odd, giving rise to his nickname, "The Horse-faced One." It is Hayagriva, you will recall, who transmitted the most powerful teachings relating to the divine Shakti Lalita in Hinduism and now those pertaining to Tara in Tantric Buddhism. If one ever thought to make a case that the celestials are really from the stars, there is likely no better collection of "proofs" than we have with Tara.

Leaving aside the more outlandish (even if intriguing) speculations of some contemporary UFOlogists, if we look to some of the stories and myths from India, Tibet, Native America, and cultures in Latin and South America, we find similarities to stories pointing to a long-standing relationship between humans on Earth and beings from somewhere else, beings that seem to want to help us advance.

Aside from Hindu myths, there are the writings of James Churchward, who spent thirty years assembling stories among the Pacific Island cultures stating that humanity and the gods came from somewhere else, "leaping onto the earth" in their present form. The plain of Nazca in South America contains ancient markings that can be recognized only from several thousand feet, presumably a signal to aircraft of some kind. Mayan drawings show strange humanlike figures lying on their backs working with instrumentation that UFOlogists have claimed are controls for an airborne craft. In October of 2000, Margalo and I were touring the Museum of Textiles in Toronto, Canada, when I spotted such a hidden drawing, intricately woven into a piece of Mayan fabric on display.

Is it the Morning Star, Tara, who shows us how far humanity can go? In the beginning of this book I described the human subtle body with its energy-processing chakras that mimic the luminous spheres of the universe. When we follow a mantra discipline, or other spiritual practice, the capacity of our chakras to process surrounding spiritual energy increases and we, even in our physical human form, take on abilities that can seem "otherworldly." We are literally evolving at a rapid rate. Is it She, along with Avalokiteshwara, Hayagriva, and others, who has been mystically leading us along? Interesting question, for which I have no answer. But after studying the legends, the questions almost pose themselves.

Mantras for Tara

The basic mantra for any anthropomorphized principle is called a *mula* or foundation mantra. The mula mantra for the great divine shakti that is Tara is given just below. In any Tibetan temple, you can hear this mantra resonating morning and evening.

Foundation Tara Mantra

1. Om Tare Tuttare Ture Swaha
[Om Tah-rei Too-tah-rei Too-rei Swah-hah]
"Om and salutations to She (Tara) who is the source of all
Blessings."

Tara Universal Peace Mantra

The mantra below asks for the great Tara energy to grant peace
to all beings.

2. Om Tare Tuttare Ture Sarva Shantim Kuru Swaha
[Om Tah-rei Too-tah-rei Too-rei Sahr-vah Shahn-teem
Koo-roo Swah-hah]
"Om and salutations to She who is the source of all bless-
ings, please bring peace to all."

Mantras for Various Types of Protection

3. Om Tare Tuttare Ture Sarva Grahe-bhyo Raksham Kuru Swaha
[Om Tah-rei Too-tah-rei Too-rei Sahr-vah Grah-hei-bhyoh
Rahk-shahm Koo-roo Swah-hah]
Protection from evil spirits

Om Tare Tuttare Ture Sarva Vighne-bhyo Raksham Kuru Swaha
[Om Tah-rei Too-tah-rei Too-rei Sahr-vah Veeg-nei-bhyoh
Rahk-shahm Koo-roo Swah-hah]
Protection from hindering forces

**Om Tare Tuttare Ture Sarva Vyadhi-bhyo Raksham
Kuru Swaha**
[Om Tah-rei Too-tah-rei Too-rei Sahr-vah Vyah-dee-bhyoh
Rahk-shahm Koo-roo Swah-hah]
Protection from diseases

**Om Tare Tuttare Ture Sarva Jware-bhyo Raksham Kuru
Swaha**
[Om Tah-rei Too-tah-rei Too-rei Sahr-vah Jwah-rei-bhyoh
Rahk-shahm Koo-roo Swah-hah]
Protection from fevers

**Om Tare Tuttare Ture Sarva Roge-bhyo Raksham Kuru
Swaha**
[Om Tah-rei Too-tah-rei Too-rei Sahr-vah Roh-gei-bhyoh
Rahk-shahm Koo-roo Swah-hah]
Protection from sickness

**Om Tare Tuttare Ture Sarva Upadrave-bhyo Raksham
Kuru Swaha**
[Om Tah-rei Too-tah-rei Too-rei Sahr-vah Oo-pah-drah-
vei-bhyoh Rahk-shahm Koo-roo Swah-hah]
Protection from injuries

**Om Tare Tuttare Ture Sarva Akalamrityu-bhyo Raksham
Kuru Swaha**
[Om Tah-rei Too-tah-rei Too-rei Sahr-vah Ah-kah-lah-
mreet-yoo-bhyoh Rahk-shahm Koo-roo Swah-hah]
Protection from untimely death

Om Tare Tuttare Ture Sarva Duh-swapnebhyo Raksham Kuru Swaha
[Om Tah-rei Too-tah-rei Too-rei Sahr-vah Doo-swahp-nei-bhyoh Rahk-shahm Koo-roo Swah-hah]
Protection from bad dreams

Om Tare Tuttare Ture Sarva Durni-mite-bhyo Raksham Kuru Swaha
[Om Tah-rei Too-tah-rei Too-rei Sahr-vah Door-nee-mee-tei-bhyoh Rahk-shahm Koo-roo Swah-hah]
Protection from evil portents

Om Tare Tuttare Ture Sarva Chitta-kule-bhyo Raksham Kuru Swaha
[Om Tah-rei Too-tah-rei Too-rei Sahr-vah Chee-tah-koo-lei-bhyoh Rahk-shahm Koo-roo Swah-hah]
Protection from confusions

Om Tare Tuttare Ture Sarva Shatru-bhyo Raksham Kuru Swaha
[Om Tah-rei Too-tah-rei Too-rei Sahr-vah Shah-troo-bhyoh Rahk-shahm Koo-roo Swah-hah]
Protection from enemies

Om Tare Tuttare Ture Sarva Bhaya-padra-vebhyo Raksham Kuru Swaha
[Om Tah-rei Too-tah-rei Too-rei Sahr-vah Bhah-yah-pah-drah-vei-bhyoh Rahk-shahm Koo-roo Swah-hah]
Protection from terrors

Om Tare Tuttare Ture Sarva Yuddeh-bhyo Raksham Kuru Swaha
[Om Tah-rei Too-tah-rei Too-rei Sahr-vah Yoo-dei-bhyoh Rahk-shahm Koo-roo Swah-hah]
Protection from battles

Om Tare Tuttare Ture Sarva Dush-krite-bhyo Raksham Kuru Swaha
[Om Tah-rei Too-tah-rei Too-rei Sahr-vah Doosh-kree-tei-bhyoh Rahk-shahm Koo-roo Swah-hah]
Protection from bad deeds

Om Tare Tuttare Ture Sarva Kritya Kakhor-debhyo Raksham Kuru Swaha
[Om Tah-rei Too-tah-rei Too-rei Sahr-vah Kreet-yah Kah-kohr-dei-bhyoh Rahk-shahm Koo-roo Swah-hah]
Protection from magical, injurious, and deadly curses

Om Tare Tuttare Ture Sarva Vise-bhyo Raksham Kuru Swaha
[Om Tah-rei Too-tah-rei Too-rei Sahr-vah Vee-sei-bhyoh Rahk-shahm Koo-roo Swah-hah]
Protection from poisons

The following English rendering of a poetic supplication shows the depth of feeling and breadth of activity accorded the Mother of Tibetan Buddhism.

Homage to Tara our Mother
  of great compassion
Homage to Tara our Mother
  a thousand hands, a thousand eyes

Homage to Tara our Mother
    queen of healers
Homage to Tara our Mother
    who conquers disease as its medicine

Homage to Tara our Mother
    who knows the means of compassion
Homage to Tara our Mother
    a foundation like the Earth

Homage to Tara our Mother
    cooling like water
Homage to Tara our Mother
    ripening like fire

Homage to Tara our Mother
    spreading like wind
Homage to Tara our Mother
    pervading everywhere like space

Protection of All

The following longish Tara mantra is commonly used as both a blessing and a purification. On one hand, it asks for purification. But the words for "crush" and "bind" also refer to those who would stand in the way of sincere aspirants. So the spirit of the mantra is also "Please help and purify me, but also stand guard against those who might oppose my progress."

4. Namo Ratna-Trayaya
Nama Arya Avalokiteshwaraya
Bodhi-sattwaya
Maha-sattwaya

Maha-karunikaya
Tad-yatha Om Tare Tuttare Ture
Sarva Dushtan Pra-dushtan
Mama Krite
Jam-bhaya Stam-bhaya Mo-haya Ban-dhaya
Hum Hum Hum Phat Phat Phat
Sarva Dushta Stam-bhani Tare Swaha

"Salutations to the three jewels (Buddha, Dharma, Sangha).
Salutation to Great Avalokiteshwara, Bodhisattva, Great
Being Greatly Compassionate; Tare Tuttare Ture all the
sins and evils I have committed, please crush, purify,
confuse, bind. Hum Hum Hum Phat Phat Phat, to Tara
who purifies all, Swaha."

Misuse of Shakti Power

In my e-mail the other day I received the following humorous bit of information on a potential application of power: "If you yelled for eight years, seven months and six days, you would have produced enough sound energy to heat one cup of coffee."

Certainly this would be a waste of a form of personal power, small though it might be. But what if you could yell once and brew your coffee? What if even that was but a small and insignificant application of the potential of the power you had within? What if you had what are called in India siddhis, a Sanskrit word for divine abilities. Although it might seem far-fetched, the huge power of shakti you possess can grant you extraordinary abilities. A little later, I'll give you examples of what I mean.

I would be remiss in this book if I did not at least touch upon the potential for the misuse of divine energy.

Any of us who practice diligently will arrive at a place where our shakti begins to respond to our conscious thoughts in powerful ways. Less well known, it is also possible that one may have done significant spiritual work in a previous life, only to have the complete fruit of that work appear in this present life in the form of a very active shakti. With an awakened shakti come gifts of power. But gifts that arrive in this way are not sealed for your protection. We still have free will. We must still make moment-to-moment decisions concerning the use of our gifts. Thus, unless a person has a solid, spiritual, and moral foundation for sudden abilities, significant problems can appear. The new reality for anyone whose shakti has been awakened is that there are now greater consequences to their actions, whether spiritual or mundane.

One of my teachers used to say, "If you ever find yourself in a situation where you feel you might do something you'd later regret, hiss like a snake but don't bite." This same teacher pointed out something that I can tell you from experience: It is not much fun to learn about misuse of energy through unwitting personal experiments.

In 1975, after several years of intense daily mantra work, I could feel that the force of shakti was beginning to respond to my thoughts and feelings. I was quite pleased with myself. One day shortly after this realization, a huge fight broke out between a couple living at our ashram. They were obviously in the breaking-up stage. After a loud muffled series of shouts from him, followed by a shriek from her, he came down the stairs as she shouted after him, "You pulled out my hair!"

Enter Thomas Ashley-Farrand, priest. Catching up with him at the back door, I said some things in the heat of anger that were as powerful as they were disparaging. I really unloaded on him. I could have said some of the same things without the negative energy I directed at him, but I did not. To my amazement, within fifteen minutes the phone rang. It was another spiritual teacher, well known to me, with a few choice words to share about the incident that, somehow, he knew about. After rebuking me, he promised that a lesson would follow. Shortly thereafter, I found that a certain spiritual gift was taken from me. The loss of it had a strongly chastening effect. Six months later, when my teacher returned to our Center for his semiannual visit, he restored the gift, confident that I had learned my lesson. I think I have.

In an earlier chapter, I told you about the disturbed woman who confronted me in Toronto. When I put up my hand in a blessing gesture and told her to be peaceful, a powerful and positive force came out of my hand and went into her. This was not something I planned, but rather the energy of my kundalini shakti responding to my peaceful intentions (all by the grace of Chamundi). If I had held a different intention or been bent on retaliation of some kind, the result may have been quite different for both of us.

In any situation where we feel moved to act, it's important that we first look for the most powerful, positive response. If an appropriate action does not seem obvious, it is probably best to do nothing until either our intuition gives us more options, or we have greater understanding.

Most spiritual leaders and teachers will find, sooner or later, that their shakti is awake in such a way that they have what must be called "spiritual authority." While this authority is a vast topic in and of itself, it is accurate to say that the effects such authority can produce in our lives are as powerful as they are profound. A teacher may affect another's karma; they can reduce it, speed its processing, or even take some piece of it upon themselves. They can effect forgiveness of karma or postpone its effects. Mundane life conditions can be altered through improved health, positive job changes, increased or accelerated spiritual growth of the student, and relationship issues can be greatly affected for the good. True spiritual teachers also can ignite the spark of developing shakti in their students and others and set them on a new course over several days, months, years, decades, or lifetimes. Anytime this level of power has been achieved, the potential exists for its corruption.

I have observed that negative applications of power are, thankfully, rare among those who have some genuine spiritual attainment. Healers of great power, such as the Christian minister Benny Hinn, are humble as they perform their good works, giving all credit to God. A nameless Hindu healer I met in the Himalayas similarly gave all credit to Shiva for his gifts of the spirit.

The powers of Satya Sai Baba are said to include the ability to materialize *vibhuti* (holy ash) and other assorted objects. Hundreds of thousands of people have witnessed these feats over years. But these materializations are not sideshow tricks. Satya Sai Baba uses his miraculous powers to inspire and uplift. Thousands of people who might not otherwise have become interested in spirituality have become attracted by his manifestations, only to find that Sai Baba's message of love and service is much more profound.

But, again, there can be a darker side, as I discovered on a trip through India in 1978.*

My trip through India took me from Cape Komorin in the south to Uttarkashi in the north. Uttarkashi, located a full day's bus trip up in the mountains from Rishikesh, is literally a town composed of swamis. Except for the occasional *bramacharya*, a celibate student or apprentice renunciate usually dressed in white, the roads are traveled by monks and swamis, creating a sea of bobbing orange robes everywhere.

When our group of Western spiritual tourists arrived in Uttarkashi, we got off the bus to some startling news. Blocked by a landslide some ten miles to the north, the flow of the Ganges River was diminishing hour by hour.

Our group of fifteen split up into five groups of three, with each group housed in separate quarters. I stayed with two other men on the second floor of a private villa in a large open room with a

*This story appears in more complete form in *True Stories of Spiritual Power* (see bibliography).

concrete floor. My roommates were a young man in his late twenties, named Darshan, and a new arrival who had joined the tour in Rishikesh. I knew nothing about the newcomer, who appeared to be in his mid-thirties. Since he was dressed in white, I assumed that he was a student of one of the swamis, an assumption I later found was incorrect.

Blankets and bedding were in ample supply, but food was another matter. As a precaution in case of further landslides and mudslides, the Indian Army Corps of Engineers had stopped all travel on the road leading back and forth between Uttarkashi and Rishikesh. Nothing came in or out of town, including food, so it was fair to assume that the dinner that was to have been prepared for us was somewhere down in the lower mountains. Not only our tour, of course, but all of Uttarkashi was short on food. When a makeshift dinner finally arrived it consisted of a stack of about ten pieces of white bread to be shared among the three of us.

Since I was near the door, Darshan, who carried the bread plate from downstairs, came to me and offered me first choice. Across the room the longhaired young man in white cleared his throat loudly. When we glanced up he vigorously motioned to Darshan to come over to him. He looked indignant and annoyed. I looked at Darshan then shrugged as he went over to the noisy throat. The loud-throated man took six pieces of the bread, and then arrogantly waved Darshan away.

In that single simple act, the young man in white taught me everything of importance about himself. He was arrogant, selfish, and self-centered. He fancied himself superior to us, and a person to be regarded as first. I found myself wondering what he was doing with us on this trip. Most of the people on this spiritual tour, although strangers at the start, were well-mannered, considerate, and sincere in their search for the truly spiritual. This fellow did not meet my personal definitions of any of these ideas. Wanting nothing at all to do with him I ate my two pieces of bread and took a nap.

Two hours later, our group assembled to go to a Sanskrit academy operated by a popular local swami. The academy was near the Ganges, which by now had slowed to a trickle. The river that normally flowed some ten feet from the outside patio was now a full hundred feet away, a slender thread of water sliding across its bed of multicolored stones and rocks. It sounded wonderfully pleasant anyway, and provided the perfect acoustical backdrop to our gathering.

The evening lecture by our host, Swami Akhandananda, focused on the topic that demonstrations of spiritual power are not to be regarded as a measure of true spiritual attainment. He spoke for some thirty minutes on this theme, ending the talk by observing that a humble attitude toward humanity, a spirit of service, and compassion for those less fortunate are what mark a truly spiritual person, and not the demonstration of whatever powers one may have accumulated along the way.

Following the lecture, it was announced, there would be a demonstration of siddhis, or divine abilities. My new roommate was introduced and strode to the front with a swagger. I could not imagine why the lecturer and the other half-dozen swamis gave this man a platform.

The young man went by the name of Shiva Bala Yogi, which means "young Shiva." I learned later that there had been a very famous man by the same name and that the young man in white had decided to adopt the name. Through an interpreter, Shiva Bala Yogi told us that when he was in his early twenties, a figure had appeared in the corner of his room one night (he had been scared half to death, he said) and gave him a blessing. From that moment thereafter, he had supernatural powers.

Then the show started.

The man announced that he would manifest vibhuti in each person's hand. Shiva Bala Yogi then rolled up his sleeves past the elbow and asked everyone to hold out his or her right hand. He moved from person to person in the group, and, rubbing his fingers together, produced ash from his fingertips in small amounts that dropped into each outstretched hand.

I had watched very carefully. With his sleeves rolled up, he could not have hidden a secret delivery tube of any kind. Still, skeptics abounded in the group. A very vocal twosome, one of whom was a college physics teacher, demanded to make an inspection. They were allowed to do so.

To make further proof of his abilities, another demonstration was demanded. Shiva Bala Yogi thought for a minute then said, "How about I bring some stones from the Ganges River. Will that satisfy you?" The group loudly assented. So again rolling up both sleeves, he went around to each person and deposited a small stone in each hand. When he got to me, I felt the stone drop into my palm from nowhere, still damp from the river. I was convinced and so was everyone else.

Shiva Bala Yogi was now puffed up with obvious pride. This posturing gave me a second window on this young man. He was actually an emotional eight- or nine-year-old, behaving as if he had never been given any instructions on the *Yamas* and *Niyamas*, spiritual "do's and don'ts," which are a reasonable Hindu approximation of the Ten Commandments or The Golden Rule.

As we were driven by bus back to our rooms for the night, the swamis and Shiva Bala Yogi stayed behind to continue their discussions about power and its relationship to true spirituality. Among our group, there was much discussion about how Bala Yogi had really come by his powers. Few believed his story of a nighttime visitation. A number felt a more plausible explanation would be that his abilities began to manifest as a result of intense discipline in a previous life, where such abilities had been ardently sought after. In this life he gave little appearance of devotion or spiritual respect to anyone or anything.

The next morning we were urgently awakened early, and told that we must get dressed, gather our belongings, and quickly board the bus. During the night the Ganges had continued to back up until it had reached a dangerously high level farther up in the Himalayas. If it backed up any more, and then broke loose uncontrolled, there would be havoc extending hundreds of miles downstream. The Indian Army Corps of Engineers had decided to blow up the blockage.

After a hastily consumed cup of tea and chapati (wheat pancake), we boarded the bus and it quickly pulled away, heading north. A mile out of town, we turned onto a well-kept dirt road that wound up, up, up, and around to a small park. There we stopped and disembarked to find ourselves three thousand feet above the bed of the Ganges below. It was show time again, though of another variety.

After about an hour an Indian army sergeant came around to make sure our group was safe and secure. He told us the blasting would take place in fifteen minutes, so we lined up on dirt banks and benches, waiting for something to happen. Exactly fifteen minutes later, the same sergeant came jogging around the corner of a hill and said the blasting had taken place and that we should see the results soon.

No matter how many times you see a spectacular sight on television, there is nothing to compare to the real thing. The scene that followed, viewed from our vantage point, looked like a toy set, but we knew it was devastatingly real.

About five to seven minutes later, we saw the first wave. A large cleft in the river's path some five miles to the north showed only a trickle of water coming through the pass. Then, suddenly, around the bend came a huge wall of turbulent brown water racing down the riverbed in boiling cascades hundreds of feet high. As it hit the flat, it spread out quickly and streamed in frothy waves toward the once placid shores.

As we watched in horrified fascination, it uprooted trees and carried them away still standing upright. Houses were lifted up and swept downstream, around a bend, and out of view. We were speechless. Soon, more houses and fences and debris of all kind showed up on the rushing river.

The swami's Sanskrit academy, where we had gathered the night before, was swept away in seconds. There was no trace of the two-story concrete structure, the accompanying dwellings, or any other items on the property. Only waves of water carrying debris.

Anything standing along the shores of the Ganges for fifty miles downstream was demolished. There were places on our route back where even the road had washed away. When we finally departed Uttarkashi later in the day, the bus could travel only a few miles before stopping. We came to places where the road was completely gone, and we were forced to walk down steep mountain embankments and then back up again to another bus waiting on the other side of the washout. That bus would ferry us another ten miles or so to the next washed-out section, and we would have to do it all over again. It took us fourteen hours to go eighty miles.

When we had safely arrived in Rishikesh, the news reached us that young Shiva Bala Yogi was dead. They had found his body washed up some twenty miles downstream from the academy. Over the next day the pieces of what had happened came together.

After we had left the gathering that night, Shiva Bala Yogi and the swamis had stayed for quite some time in animated dialogue, debating what is spiritual and what is not. Shiva Bala Yogi was so incensed that the swamis did not give him respect for his abilities that at the end of their talks he had uttered the Hindi equivalent of "I'll show you all" and stalked off. Walking about three hundred yards down the Ganges from where we had all gathered, he found a secluded spot, sat down, and assumed the classic yogic posture. There, he entered a deep meditative state.

When the warnings had come the following morning, his consciousness was nowhere near a place or in a state where he could hear and respond to them. He was still deep in meditation with his body essentially parked until he returned to it. When the river came rushing down, it had picked up his body and carried it away. It was still in a yogic posture when recovered hours later. His powers had not protected him from death. According to the swamis who were present the evening before and heard about his death, he had intended to leave his body and then perform some miraculous event to shame or humiliate them, thereby proving his superiority. Mother Nature, it seemed, had another plan.

Shiva Bala Yogi's spiritual powers, however they may have been acquired, were quite real as far as any of us could tell. But since he had no formal training in the positive use of his gifts or the penalty for misuse, he just used them to satisfy his own ego and pride.

As Swami Akhandananda pointed out so poignantly, demonstrations of spiritual abilities are not an accurate indication of the level of anyone's true spiritual development. Our everyday behavior is the ultimate determinator. Overt behavior in the form of action, and covert behavior in the form of thoughts, prayers, devotion to ideals, lofty objectives for self and others, all inevitably reveal spiritual status. Behavior that promotes the essential unity of humanity through positive means is a clear indication of spiritual advancement or attainment. Anything else is either misuse of power or irrelevant, spiritually speaking. As pointless as trying to heat up a cup of coffee by yelling.

If we dedicate our actions to service to God through humanity, we should never have to worry about misusing the awakened shakti. The great ones in the world's religions have demonstrated the spirit of service to others in any miracle attributed to them. Jesus, for example, is quoted as saying to those around him, "And greater things shall you do." I do not for a moment think that he was referring only to his disciples. Throughout his brief public mission, he continually demonstrated that power, even such great power as he possessed, has only one true spiritual purpose: service.

At times it may be that even if we attempt to live in the spirit of service we are unsure as to whether our actions are appropriate to a given situation. One of my teachers used to recommend that we pray for guidance and then act on intuition. "Put forth your best efforts, then leave the rest to God," he would say. There is another old saying in spiritual circles that states with simplicity, "Sincerity invokes protection." If one makes mistakes with the best of intentions, karmic results are often mitigated.

Although the exact mechanism of this mitigation is not known, I suspect the grace of Divine Mother herself. For if all actions are the result of her power acting through us in some way, then she also has authority over karmic results of use of her power.

Shakti and Your Life

The more that shakti manifests in your life, the more your life will change. Whether it is in the area of relationships, health, employment, family and children, or something else altogether, circumstances in your everyday existence will be altered. For some, such changes began a number of years ago with the appearance of gurus from India and later Tibet. For others, attraction to a spiritual teacher did not begin until the teachers began to appear in a feminine form.

Women Gurus in Modern Times

In the years before the change over to the new millennium, numerous powerful feminine spiritual teachers and gurus began to appear seemingly quite suddenly. The shakti power inherent in both the new age and in women manifested the immediate appearance of advanced spiritual teachers who are women. While the following descriptions of such teachers are representative, they are by no means intended to be complete or comprehensive.

Daya Mata, a disciple of Paramahansa Yogananda and one of the first women spiritual leaders to appear in the West, has been the spiritual leader of the Self-Realization Fellowship since the 1960s. Promulgating the teachings of Yogananda through his international best-seller *Autobiography of a Yogi* and other works, she has followed the instructions of Yogananda in teaching the ancient Kriya Yoga techniques to a Western audience.

Although she never used the title herself, Earlyne Chaney, co-founder of Astara, who left her body in 1997, was widely regarded by her followers as a guru. Starting in 1980, she held annual fire initiation ceremonies that drew more than a thousand people from all over the world. She and her husband, Robert Chaney, would receive each spiritual aspirant seeking initiation in a ceremony often lasting from 7:00 P.M. until 4:00 in the morning. Her shakti was powerfully awake, and she used it to uplift and inspire thousands of seekers during fifty years of service.

Gurumayi, leader of the Siddha Yoga Foundation, is a disciple of Paramahansa Muktananda, a popular and well-known guru from India who traveled widely in the 1970s. She received his spiritual mantle before he left his body and has run the organization he founded since 1982. She visits Siddha Yoga centers in many major cities every year, holding satsang (divine discussion) and giving initiations. In those centers, you can hear devotees chanting the great siddha mantra "Om Namah Shivaya" long into the night.

Sakya Jetsun Chiney Luding, called Jetsun Ma, is a Tibetan teacher who visited Los Angeles in the early 1980s. Traveling from her home in Vancouver twice a year, she gave a variety of classical Tibetan Buddhist empowerments. Born into a royal family, she began her spiritual studies at the age of eight and continued her studies until forced to flee Tibet. Her brother is the prominent Tibetan spiritual leader H. H. Sakya Trizin Jetsun Kusho.

More recently, others have come into prominence. Ammachi, a woman from India with increasing popularity, is known as the "hugging guru." People line up in long queues wherever she appears, and Ammachi patiently hugs each and every devotee who comes before her. She has probably logged more hugs in the last five years than all the rest of the gurus combined. In a world where love is needed so much, hers is a powerful message and a wonderfully positive contribution to Western spirituality.

Early in 1997, Sadguru Sant Keshavadas gave his wife, Rama Mata, *guru diksha* (initiation) on the banks of the Ganges River and changed her name to Guru Mata. In December of that year he left his body. Now Guru Mata presides over the Sanatana Vishwa Dharma organization he founded in 1973 from international headquarters in Bangalore, India. In this country the organization is called Cosmic Religion. She travels to the United States every year for programs. Her spiritual authority is often hidden by her great humility.

The last several years have seen the emergence of Karunamayi, a guru also from Bangalore, who, followers claim, is an emanation of Saraswati. Like the more famous Satya Sai Baba, Karunamayi manifests vibhuti and other objects before small groups of followers to inspire them on their spiritual path. She teaches mantra practices and often performs the Lalita Puja or the ceremony propitiating "She with a thousand names and powers," discussed in Chapter 9. Karunamayi travels to the United States each year to teach, initiate students, and conduct Vedic ceremonies.

Sri Anandi Ma is a guru of the Kundalini Maha Yoga lineage who offers cassettes and CDs through Sounds True. Although little known in the United States, her students here are dedicated and ardently practice disciplines given by her.

Shree Ma, Holy Mother from Kamakhya in Assam, is the guru of American-born Swami Satyananda Saraswati. Inspired by her, he has published books on the ancient ceremonies of India, including the comprehensive works *Chandi Path* and *Kali Puja*. The energy of the Great Feminine permeates Swami Satyananda's works, who in turn gives the credit to his guru, Shree Ma.

There is one more woman who may have been on your mind as she has been on mine, Mother Teresa of Calcutta. She probably would not call herself a guru but more of a Christian disciple following the model of St. Francis. But she did exhibit some of the characteristics of a guru. First, she has disciples. The order of nuns that formed around her has spread over the globe as women in blue-and-white habits pledge themselves to the joyful service of those who are very ill or preparing to leave the Earth plane. Second, she was able to pass energy through chakras in her hands.

I first observed her passing energy to others while I was watching television. She picked up an infant and, cupping her hand oddly, slapped it on the back. I sat up straight in my chair, probably with my mouth agape. Then she waited, looked at the baby, and did it again. I could sense quite plainly that she was sending prana and perhaps spiritual electricity into the child. The next time I saw her pass energy, the pope was on the receiving end. Shown in a television meeting with Pope John Paul I, she kissed his ring then slapped his palm the same way she had slapped the infant. Then she roared with laughter. So did I when I saw it. She sent him some juice, probably hoping it might help him stay around a little longer.

These are but a few of the women gurus of whom I am aware. There are surely many others, engaged in humble service. I salute them all.

Looking Forward

I suggest to you that as we move further into the Aquarian energy, more and more people will receive gifts of the spirit. Viewed from an Eastern perspective, the power of shakti will move in us more powerfully than ever before, and those who have been preparing to receive this power will find more resources than they ever would have dreamed of just thirty years ago. There are those among us who will suddenly become spiritual teachers with a stature we have only seen from our Indian and Tibetan friends. Indeed, they have been diligently preparing us for that eventuality for many years, some for lifetimes.

Not all those who have these resources will be schooled in the Eastern methods. Whether Christian, Jew, Muslim, Native Shaman, or other, those following any genuine path with sincerity and dedication will see significant changes in themselves. More healers, true spiritual teachers and initiators, psychics, and those who manifest miraculous things will appear among us than ever before. Most of them will be sincere and service-oriented.

Shakti Pushes and We Move

Throughout this work I have presented mantra formulas for your use framed in the context of stories and myths, primarily from India. The characters and the plots were fables. The mantra powers contained in the stories and the power of the kundalini shakti sitting at the base of your spine area are real.

As you practice Sanskrit mantra and grow in proficiency, you will obtain the effects you desire. After all, that is why you did them in the first place. But there will be other effects that follow the first ones. When you experience results, you will decide that there are more conditions you would like to change, or more effects you desire to create, so you will perform more disciplines with mantra. By that time, you will grow to appreciate the inflow of energy. At some subtle level, you will understand that your overall store of spiritual energy is increasing as your spiritual bulb increases its wattage. Now Divine Mother has you. By showing you the increase in energy, She will motivate you to further efforts. By solving your problems and fulfilling your desires, She will move you down the road to spiritual advancement. Like any good mother, she will pack your lunch with the finest fruit and sandwiches, then send you off to advance in the school of life. As you begin to make your way with these new tools, your life will undergo subtle changes.

Here are some statements about the movement of shakti within us. One or more of them may seem quite familiar.

- When shakti moves within, it is the Great Feminine trying to get our attention.
- When shakti moves within, our entire lives can change. There may be great upheavals that occur from nowhere. They can be disconcerting, maddening, frustrating, joyful, and life-altering, but they always move us forward.
- When shakti moves within, we must often shift from our comfortable positions (physical, emotional, and mental) or suffer some consequence until an important lesson is learned.
- When shakti moves within, the extent of our ignorance about spiritual things is made abundantly clear.
- The movement of shakti within cannot be stopped, but it can be redirected. We may have no choice but to heed its call, but choices among the paths emerging from our decisions still remain.
- The movement of shakti within inevitably leads to both Love and Knowledge, in this or a subsequent life. The Great Feminine is loving and giving by nature. Therefore, we must assume She is trying to give us something new that She thinks we need.

- When shakti moves within, the Great Feminine has blessed us in a momentous way.
- When shakti moves within, Divine Grace is at hand.

But if shakti moves within us, where will it ultimately lead?

- Shakti leads to the Divine Beloved within, where all questions are answered, all tears are dried, where all Love resides, all Knowledge is contained.
- Shakti leads to true Self-knowledge. Knowing oneself leads to knowing others as well.
- Shakti leads to contact with the higher levels of reality, such as the realms where the Great Ones and the celestials reside.
- Shakti leads to the end of the round of rebirth, producing true liberation.
- Shakti leads to the doorway, passing through which one leaves behind all realms, both physical and nonphysical.

What Will You Do?

Near the end of *Healing Mantras*, I posed a question that bears repeating here: What will you do once you have finally fulfilled your desires? Will you then pursue other desires? What will you do if you discover you have real power? If all power is transitory and ephemeral, what effects do you want to leave behind, both within and without?

While we are each individuals, we are also one. That which binds us together is love. It seems to me the important question becomes: How can you achieve a state of Love other than by loving? Will you pray over what actions to take? Not getting what may seem to you to be a satisfactory response from prayer, will you make decisions that just seem true and correct and proceed anyway? Are you prepared to take responsibility for your decisions and actions, no matter what? Is there any other potential choice than taking such responsibility anyway? The answers to these questions will determine your fate over many lives.

I have only one suggestion based upon my experiments and my experience. Leave everything to God first, last, and always. If you have some real power or have it given to you, dedicate its use to the service of others. Having made such a foundation decision, put forth your best efforts and leave the rest to the divine. If you even attempt to do this, you will actually escape the results of some mistakes you might make along the way.

As I said in Chapter 11, you can make honest mistakes while trying to serve with complete sincerity and be spared the karmic return of such mistakes. Sincerity is like a shield against karmic return from mistakes. Such is the compassion of God, the Masters, the celestials, and the Great Ones who walk among us. Even if our mistakes cause the necessity of some kind of karmic return, even if the mistakes are great and the negative result great, sometimes the Great Ones will take the effects upon themselves. They know they can handle it or neutralize it better than we can. When Jesus was crucified, it is said he died for our sins. Was this not taking the karma of humanity upon himself? Unknown spiritual teachers of high stature and the Great Ones have been doing such things for centuries. Maybe a time will come when you can add your shoulder to the wheel and help push along humanity's seemingly slow, painful trek to its birthright of divinity.

Finally, there is nothing at all wrong with making changes in your life for the better. You are entitled to all the good things you can bring to yourself, your family, your friends, and your community. In the process, help to make the ultimate manifestation of your shakti rest on a foundation of Divine Love. It is our common human destiny. So make a decision to affirm your own nature as one of Divine Love, using the mantra,

Aham Prema
[Ah-hahm Preh-mah]
"I am Divine Love."

She who empowers all, in every realm, will surely respond.

Using Mantras in a Spiritual Practice

To help you plan a mantra discipline for helping yourself or others, this appendix will discuss the mechanics of mantra practice designed to accomplish a specific goal. There are two different categories of mantra disciplines that have been taught for centuries.

Forty-Day Approach

Write down on a slip of paper what it is you are trying to accomplish. Fold the paper and put it in a special place for the duration of your discipline. For the next forty days repeat your mantra during twice-daily sessions lasting from ten to thirty minutes, preferably in the morning and evening. If you are able, use the same place for your mantra practice throughout your discipline. At any time during the forty days, you may take out your piece of paper to help you focus on your goal, then return it to its place. When the forty-day period is complete, light a candle and burn the paper, feeling that you are offering the idea on the paper to your own divine self and to God. Now wait for the results, although you may already be seeing changes in the circumstances that are the subject of your discipline.

If your karma related to the subject of your discipline is particularly troublesome, it may take more than one such discipline. One man, whom I'll call Jack, was determined to improve his business. He undertook a Lakshmi discipline with intensity but reaped no noticeable result upon finishing. Undeterred, he completed a second discipline, also with very little result. Still pursuing his objective, he performed a third discipline with a Lakshmi mantra and the floodgates opened. He later told me that at some level he knew all along that he was working through karma in the area of his finances. Jack is a superb example of the spirit and stamina needed to approach any discipline. He had faith in the method as well as faith in himself. He was diligent, dedicated, and did not give up. In just 120 days, he worked through his karma relating to finances and changed his life.

Mantra Siddhi

There is a mysterious relationship between the heart and shakti. Over a sustained period of time of chanting mantras, the power of the mantra comes to rest in the heart, even as it reverberates in the mind while energizing the chakras. When this happens, a mystical resonance takes place in the shakti at the base of the spine. Providing the energy for manifestation for that which resides in the heart, the shakti empowers the heart's desire expressed through the mind.

Because results of mantra practice were closely watched over many years in India, specific standards of achievement came to be linked to a certain number of repetitions. It became apparent that 125,000 mantra repetitions were required to seat a mantra in the heart. While this figure is not ironclad, it is a very close approximation to what you can expect. This number of repetitions will enable you to reach what is called Mantra Siddhi, a term denoting power and facility with the mantra. More repetitions magnify the result even more, so that one may affect not only one's own life but others as well. By prayer combined with mantra, for example, you can chant mantra on behalf of others. But always preface such work with the prayer that while you are doing this for so and so's benefit, you are not taking their karma.

Because I teach mantra, I have made it a personal requirement to seek Mantra Siddhi for a wide variety of mantras. This enables me to be of greater aid to others than if I worked with only one or two mantras. If you have a desire to teach mantra disciplines, I recommend this approach highly.

Beads and Malas

Many mantra disciplines employ a mala, which is a Hindu form of the rosary that precedes the Catholic rosary by several thousand years. Most malas have either 54 beads (half mala), like the Catholic rosary, or 108 beads, which is called a full mala. The reason 108 beads are used is directly tied to the number of energy channels, nadis, surrounding the spiritual heart in the subtle body. As each mantra is chanted, energy is invoked into one channel so that by completion of the round of chanting on the mala, energy has passed into all of the 108 nadis that surround the spiritual heart.

Beads used in malas come from many sources. Sandalwood is the most common, followed by Tulasi (basil, said to be attuned to Vishnu) and Rudraksha (said to be attuned to Shiva and Kali or Durga). Rudraksha beads are reputed to have a powerful healing effect on the user or wearer. In each case, the wood or berry is dried, drilled, and strung.

A single bead, called the *meru* (mountain in Sanskrit) is designated as the beginning and ending point for repetitions and is fastened as a separate bead. When chanting while using a mala, begin with the bead right next to the meru, and chant on each bead, moving along the mala by pushing beads with your thumb and index finger. Eventually, you will chant a mantra for each bead on the mala and arrive back at the meru bead. Do not cross the meru bead. Instead, begin pushing each bead away as you chant each mantra. The meru stores a portion of the energy of chanting so that over time it gains a strong vibration. This is why you will often see practitioners wearing a necklace of beads. They want the power of their chanting to accompany them wherever they go.

Malas can be purchased at many spiritual bookstores and online.

Glossary

Acupuncture System and spiritual science of placing tiny needles in the human physical body to optimize the flow of vital energy in the subtle body, with healing or better health as the goal.

Ajna Chakra Spiritual center between the eyebrows, often referred to as the sixth chakra, where the masculine and feminine currents in the body meet and join. The merging of the two currents produce an interior sound, "Om."

Anasuya Enlightened wife of Sage Atri and mother of the first guru, Dattatreya. It is unclear whether Dattatreya (technically adopted by his parents) is mythical or actually lived thousands of years ago.

Aquarius The eleventh sign of the zodiac. An age lasting 2,000 years thought by many to have begun in the year 2001.

Archetype Fundamental symbol or representation, sometimes given human form and attributes for the purpose of making certain concepts easier to understand and remember.

Astrology Study of the movement of the planets and the effect of their vibrations in human events and behavior. The Eastern system is Moon-centered while the Western system is Sun-centered.

Atri Ancient sage considered one of the great Rishis of ancient India. He and his wife, Anasuya, had an understanding of the transcendental nature of Lakshmi that goes far beyond simple prosperity.

Aura Spiritual light around every living thing. Some people have the ability to see this light as a generalized halo, while others see different colors, usually around human beings.

Avatar A divine being with no karma whatsoever who comes to Earth to perform specific beneficial tasks for humanity. There are many varieties and types of avatars.

Bhakti Yoga The Yoga of Devotion to God. Highest states are Prema—Divine Love and Prapatti—total surrender, and faith in God's benevolent activity.

Brahma Personified Vedic god representative of the known universe and all of its contents. Also called the creator of the universe in ancient story-based scriptures called the Puranas.

Brahmanas Scriptures that preceded the Upanishads which are said to be summaries of the Brahmanas.

Brahmin The priest class and highest caste in India.

Buddha The Ninth Avatar of Vishnu. Also, a state of consciousness.

Daksha Father of Parvati (also called Sati, Hemavati, and other names).

Devi Feminine celestial spirit or entity.

Dhanvantari The celestial healer who appeared at the churning of the ocean of consciousness just as Lakshmi did. He distributed the Nectar of Immortality while giving discourse on the healing properties of plants, gems, and other remedies.

Durga Personified feminine power of protection. Member of the Hindu feminine trinity.

Durvasas A son of Sage Atri and his enlightened wife, Anasuya. He is depicted as very powerful, a bit stern, and not known for his forbearance.

Etheric Body A subtle energy body interpenetrating the physical body. It is in the etheric body that the chakras are found. Sometimes referred to as the astral body.

Feminine Trinity Traditionally Lakshmi, Saraswati, and Durga.

Ganges River in India said to remove sins of many lives in a single bathing.

Gayatri The feminine name given to the spiritual energy that comes to Earth through the sun from the higher realms. It is a personification of spiritual light. Also, a particular rhythm or cadence given to a class of mantras.

Gayatri Mantra A spiritual formula for bringing in or increasing the flow of spiritual light into oneself, often called The Essence of the Vedas.

This mantra on universal spiritual light and sound is practiced by Hindus of every caste and some branches of Buddhism that work with mantra.

Granthis Spiritual knots, three in number, located along the spine in the subtle body that prevent premature entrance of kundalini energy into centers on the spine above the sacral center (Swadhisthana Chakra). Were this energy to travel up the spine before the spiritual vehicle is ready, harm to the physical body could result.

Guru Literally, "that which dispels darkness." In this case, it is the darkness of ignorance. Although many teachers hold that the true guru is not a person but a principle, the term "guru" is often used colloquially to denote an advanced spiritual teacher (also see Upaguru). An enlightened spiritual teacher with the ability to transmit spiritual energy by one or more methods.

Hatha Yoga The branch of yoga that practices physical movements and postures designed to prepare the body to receive kundalini energy as it moves up the spine.

Hemavati Another name for Parvati.

Iccha Shakti The Power of Will, manifesting as the power behind muscle movement, as well as the power to accomplish tasks.

Indra Chief of the celestials. In the Puranas (story-based Hindu scriptures), Indra is the one who leads the celestials in battle against their arch rivals the Asuras.

Jnana Spiritual knowledge.

Jnana Shakti The power to understand both spiritual and mundane subjects. Governs memory as well as the power of the mind to analyze perceptual and other data and information on any subject.

Kala Sanskrit for "time."

Kalachakra An esoteric chakra located above the heart center but below the throat center. Literally, the "Wheel of Time." The Kalachakra deity of Tibetan Buddhism is a concrete symbol for the interplay of time, represented by a conjoining of masculine and feminine beings or parts of the same being. This masculine-feminine joining is called yub-yum in Tibetan Buddhism. Also called the Lalani Chakra.

Kalachakra Mantra A Tibetan spiritual formula for transcending and mastering the concept of time. It eventually produces Siddhis similar to those on the Siddha Path in Hinduism.

Kali The most unbridled and raw form of personified feminine power in Hinduism.

Kali Yuga Spiritual Winter. This time period, lasting 432,000 years, began just over 5,000 years ago according to calculations based upon data in the Mahabharata. This date for the inception of Kali Yuga is used by the Brahmin priest class, the Shankaracharyas, and other Hindu spiritual authorities.

Kama Desire. In the mythic Hindu stories, Kama is similar to Cupid.

Karma The law of cause and effect. The sum total of actions and thoughts that cause a reaction or return of like energy to the source that generated it. Reincarnation or rebirth continues until all karma is balanced or neutralized. Sanchita Karma: The total of all karma from all lifetimes. Prarabdha Karma: Planetary karma represented by the natal birth chart in a particular birth or incarnation. Agami Karma: Returning karma from this and other lifetimes. Kriyamana Karma: Immediate results from present actions.

Karma Yoga The Yoga of Action. In this practice, every action is dedicated to the divine. Thus detachment is developed in the midst of all daily activities.

Kaustubha Gem Literally "Wish-fulfilling Gem." It is a spiritual condition of advanced adepts that allows what they think or speak to manifest as a blessing.

Kavacha Spiritual armor, usually built through repetition of mantra formulas designed to produce protection.

Kriya Shakti The Power of Manifestation. The very creation of the universe is said to be a manifestation of Kriya Shakti, personified by Lakshmi.

Kriya Yoga Form of yoga employing meditation and certain pranayama and mantra practices. Popularized in the West by Paramahansa Yogananda.

Kundalini The coiled, serpentine feminine energy lying in repose at the base of the human spine. Although powering all activities in the physical and subtle bodies, it is still characterized as dozing or being asleep in most people. When it awakens, new spiritual abilities manifest in individuals. Eventually it moves as an energy force up the spine in the subtle body, usually over more than one lifetime, until it reaches the crown chakra at the top of the head. At each chakra located along the spine, it releases energy leading to increased spiritual knowledge and abilities. Once the energy has reached the top of the head, one becomes "Shiva" and is liberated from the necessity of rebirth, although one may choose rebirth for the purpose of service to mankind. All forms of shakti may manifest: Kriya, Jnana, Iccha, Para, and Mantra, to name but a few.

Kundalini Shakti The category of shakti that balances one's birth situation with karma. Electricity (both spiritual and mundane) and magnetism are manifestations of this power.

Kundalini Yoga Yoga practices that have as their objective the controlled awakening of the kundalini energy.

Lakshmana Rama's younger brother who traveled with him when Rama was banished to the forest for fourteen years.

Lakshmi The creative power of Narayana. Spouse of Vishnu and also the shakti of Shiva, according to the Maha Lakshmi Astakam. Popularly, the goddess of fortune and prosperity.

Lalita She of a thousand powers. Tantric master Hayagriva and his great student Agastya promulgated this system of working with the elements of nature. Tantra means working consciously with the obvious and subtle powers available in the universe.

Lama Tibetan monk.

Laya Yoga Yoga that achieves its goal by dissolving into the supreme through mantra, pranayama, or both.

Lotus A type of flower that grows in muck and mud. This fact is used as symbolism for the flower of spiritual progress, which can grow from the muck of even the worst karma. Often used as a reference to the heart's lotus or chakra.

Maha Great. Also a spiritual plane (Maha Loka) in the nonphysical universe where sages and saints of high attainment are said to dwell.

Maha Kalpa Great Age. The number of years the universe will last. Many ancient spiritual sources agree that this number is 311,040,000,000,000 years.

Manipura Chakra The third chakra, located at the solar plexus.

Manjushri Bodhisattva of wisdom and knowledge, usually shown holding the sword of discriminating wisdom. Tibetan spouse of Saraswati.

Mantra Shakti The power of mantra to awaken in the sayer abilities relative or pertaining to the other major categories of shakti power.

Mantra Siddhi The power one attains when one has unwrapped the power of the mantra through repetition. Mantra Siddhi is generally recognized as beginning at 125,000 repetitions of a mantra, and increases as more repetitions are completed.

Masculine Trinity Brahma, Vishnu, and Shiva in classical Hinduism.

Menaka Parvati's mother.

Mount Kailas Mountain in the Himalayas where Shiva is said to dwell.

Nadis Astral nerve tubes, similar to veins, that run through the subtle body.

Nandi A bull who is the vehicle of Shiva.

Narayana Personification of the source of all of this reality, including the creation of Brahma the Creator. Also concurrently, the threefold flame burning in the Hrit Padma. This seeming duality is intended to demonstrate that we may seem parted but are never really separated from God or the Divine.

Para Supreme. Also silent or unmanifest speech. This is the silent speech that some may hear in silence. Sages communicate by this method and adepts are heard by their teachers and masters. Ultimately, this is the most powerful form of speech. Because of the background "chatter" common to the lower mind, this divine speech can be confused with forms that only imitate it. Only advanced spiritual discrimination can tell the difference.

Para Shakti Literally, supreme shakti. As a category of shakti, its domain is heat and light—both spiritual and material. Thus, the enlightened ones have invoked Para Shakti in one of its fullest spiritual manifestations while still in the body.

Paramahansa The supreme swan. The swan here is another name for the self in the Hrit Padma. Paramahansa is a title given to a person who has demonstrated exceptionally high spiritual attainment. In modern times, Paramahansa Muktananda, Paramahansa Yogananda, and Paramahansa Ramakrishna are well-known examples.

Parvati Spouse of Shiva. In other guises she is also Durga, Kali, and Chamundi.

Pashyanti The power of sound in its intuitive form. Whispering or muttering mantras (called Pashyanti) work primarily through the second chakra.

Prana A life force that exists in the subtle body. There are five divisions of this life force. *Prana:* Situated in the region of the heart, this energy moves the lungs for inhalation and exhalation. *Apana:* This energy, situated below the navel, is associated with elimination of spent energy and waste products from the physical body. *Vyana:* This energy pervades the whole body and gives rise to the sense of touch. *Udana:* An energy centered in the throat that provides connection and disconnection of the mind from the body during deep sleep or when engaged in advanced yogic practices. It does this by closing off the throat chakra while leaving a chord or strand attached to the traveling subtle body. *Samana:* This energy at the navel center digests food and distributes the energy derived to all parts of the body, permeating the subtle body equally in every part.

Puranas Indian prehistory, myth, and stories all mixed up together. Vast amounts of spiritual information and teachings exist in the hundreds of Puranas that still exist.

Radha Krishna's lover when he was a cowherd lad.

Raja Yoga Royal path of yoga consisting of the threefold practice of Jnana, Bhakti, and Karma Yogas.

Rama Seventh Avatar of Vishnu. He came to show how potential nobility can actually manifest. He was the perfect ruler, husband, sage, friend, and brother.

Ravana Second incarnation of Jaya (of Jaya and Vijaya, gatekeepers of Narayana) in which he and his brother are nearly unconquerable demons. The only way for divine order to be restored on earth is for an incarnation of Vishnu to appear. Thus, Rama took embodiment and slew him.

Rukmini Spouse of Krishna. Some say that she and Radha are the same being.

Sadguru A God-realized teacher beyond the realms of energy-identified existence or mind-identified existence. A being firmly established in a form of enlightened activity that appears similar to daily human life. The sadguru has a specific job of leading souls to spiritual freedom. Sadgurus have no karma in the normal sense of the word. Any seeming karma, called "Yoga Yoga Samsaras," is created by sadgurus to help hide their true nature and aid their work.

Sage Narada A sage created at the time the universe came into being. He is said to be welcome everywhere and know the spiritual practices of the people wherever he goes. Always traveling, he is also said to stir things up spiritually, with the goal of bringing people closer to divine truth. Sage that brought the great Satya Narayana Puja to planet Earth.

Sahaja Samadhi Divine absorption in the midst of daily life. The infrequent sadgurus among humanity operate from this state of consciousness.

Samadhi Mind merged, absorbed in the divine. There are several types of Samadhi. With form, where one is merged with a form of the divine beloved. Formless, where the meditator is one with the great principles that formed and operate the universe at all levels.

Sanjivani Mantra This secret mantra is said to have the power to raise the dead when one has achieved its siddhi.

Saraswati Personified feminine energy for the arts, music, sciences, spiritual pursuits, and knowledge of all kinds.

Sati Another name for Parvati.

Satyabhama Krishna's second queen. Rukmini is the first.

Shakti Power, or personification of power. Personification is used in myths and stories to make complex ideas easier to understand.

Shiva Personification of consciousness in a male form. This personification is used in myths and stories to make complex ideas easier to understand.

Siddhi A seemingly magical spiritual ability or gift. Plural is siddhis.

Sita Lakshmi come in the form of Rama's wife during his tenure on Earth.

Sri Vidya Literally the shakti that gives knowledge. Sri signifies shakti and Vidya means specific knowledge (as apart from Jnana which means more generalized knowledge). The term is most often associated with Saraswati and Lalita. In Tantric disciplines, Sri Vidya is a fifteen-syllabled mantra of great power. It almost never appears in print and is usually passed on from teacher to student.

Subrahmanya Son of Shiva and Parvati. Some stories place his birth prior to Ganesha while others place it later. Esoterically, Subrahmanya consciousness is the highest possible stage of consciousness while still identified as an individual. The next step is merging in the divine in which there is no "self and other." Only unity exists.

Swadhisthana Chakra The second chakra, located at the genital center.

Tantra Means of working with the energy of nature, including the elements that rule the chakras: earth, water, fire, air, and ether. One of the most famous Tantric masters was the legendary Padmasambhava from northern India who responded to the Buddhist call for help in Tibet after Buddhism had been defeated by the Bon Po priests indigenous to Tibet. Another great Tantric Master was Hayagriva who taught in both India and Tibet. Historically, this term is sometimes associated with sexual union without climax to achieve movement of the kundalini up the spine. Although widely understood in this context in the West, such practices were used in only a handful of temples and rarely worked effectively to achieve its stated spiritual goals.

Tummo A practice producing intense body heat. Tibetan monks are preeminent in this practice during which wet sheets are dried while the practitioner sits in cold or snow.

Uddhava Friend of Krishna who, although possessed of supreme wisdom, was a butcher—lower than even a sudra in old India. His great teaching, the Uddhava Gita, is said to be outshone only by the Bhagavad Gita of Krishna.

Uma Another name for Parvati, spouse of Shiva.

Upaguru Literally, "the enlightener without form." The omnipresent "teacher without form" that can manifest in seemingly bizarre ways. It can appear as "the magazine article that seems like it was written just for you, " or "a statement by an actor in a televised drama that is so powerful for you that it nearly brings you out of your chair." These are examples of how the upaguru, a principle residing in everyone, may teach and lead.

Upamshu This is the sound that is spoken. In this state, it has a powerful effect on the physical body. Karma is reduced. Negative conditions are very positively affected.

Upanishads A series of scriptures that are all that remains of a much larger, older body of scriptures. Originally written on palm leaves many centuries ago, the number of scriptures became so unwieldy that they were summarized. Some Upanishads are actually summaries of summaries.

Vach Spiritual speech. An ancient name for Saraswati.

Varuna The presiding spirit over water. Whether the ocean, river, pond, or bathtub, the spirit is the same.

Vedanta The study of the Vedas and other spiritual texts of "revelations." Understanding of the nature of this reality and self-realization are the goals of Vedanta.

Vedas The world's oldest extant scriptures originating in India: Rig Veda, Yejur Veda, Sama Veda, and Artharva Veda. Beginning shortly after the advent of writing, increasingly stores of spiritual literature and information were summarized as the years went by. The Vedas were considered so important that they were never summarized.

Vedic Pertaining to the Vedas.

Vibhuti Holy ash, usually materialized by an adept.

Vidya Specific knowledge in a definitive category often denoted by another word preceding Vidya.

Vishnu The Vedic god of preservation. It is said that all true spiritual leaders and teachers from any religion carry the energy of Vishnu.

Vishwamitra Sage who, when he became a Brahma Rishi through the grace of Brahma Rishi Vasista, heard the rhythms of the self-luminous spheres of light in the form of the Gayatri Mantra, which makes him the seer of this universal mantra for spiritual illumination.

Yajna Sacrifice, usually in the sense of a ritual fire worship ceremony in which negative karma can be consumed or transmuted.

Yoga Literally "union" as it applies to union with the divine. There are many varieties and types of yoga, each with it's philosophic approach and specific practices.

Yoga Sutras of Patanjali A text on various yogic methods, practices, and their fruits. Alternately a manual of practices and a philosophical treatise, this work is both practical and instructive. There are many differing translations and interpretations of various sections of this work by the sage Patanjali.

Yuga Spiritual Age, or period of time in the life of the universe. There are Yugas and Maha Yugas. Here is a short summary:

Winter (Kali Yuga)	432,000 years
Spring (Treta Yuga)	1,296,000 years
Summer (Satya or Krita Yuga)	1,728,000 years
Autumn (Dwapara Yuga)	864,000 years
One Complete Yuga Revolution (Mahayuga)	4,320,000 years

It continues from there: 1,000 revolutions is a Manvantara and is 4,320,000,000 years long. This amount of time is also called a Day in the Life of Brahma. It is followed by a Night of equal length. Three hundred sixty days and nights of Brahma are called One Year of Brahma. One hundred such years constitute the life of this universe, or a Maha Kalpa—311,040,000,000,000 years.

There is also a short 24,000-year cycle in which the axis of the earth spends 2,000 years in each sign of the zodiac. It is this cycle that astrologers are referring to when they say that we are in the Age of Aquarius.

Bibliography

Ann, Martha, and Dorothy Myers Imel. *Goddesses in World Mythology.* Santa Barbara, Calif.: ABC-CLIO, Inc., 1993.

Ashley-Farrand, Thomas. *Healing Mantras.* New York: Ballantine Wellspring Books, 1999.

———. *The Ancient Science of Sanskrit Mantra and Ceremony:* vol. I, *Mantra;* vol. 2, *Mantras and Great Spiritual Disciplines;* and vol. 3, *Ceremonies.* Privately published, 1995–9; available at www.sanskritmantra.com.

———. *True Stories of Spiritual Power.* Privately published, 1995; available at www.sanskritmantra.com.

Avalon, Arthur (pen name of Sir John Woodroffe). *Tantra of the Great Liberation.* New York: Dover Publications, Inc., 1972.

Bachofen, J. J. *Myth, Religion & Mother Right,* trans. Ralph Manheim. New York: Princeton/Bollingen, 1973.

Beyer, Stephen. *The Cult of Tara.* Los Angeles and Berkeley: University of California Press, 1978.

Blavatsky, H. P. *The Secret Doctrine.* Pasadena, Calif.: Theosophical University Press, (1888) 1970.

Blofeld, John. *Bodhisattva of Compassion: The Mystical Tradition of Kuan Yin.* Boston: Shambhala Publications, Inc., 1988.

———. *Mantras: Sacred Words of Power.* New York: E. P. Dutton, 1977.

Board of Scholars. *Mantramahoddadhi.* Delhi, India: Sri Satguru Publications, 1984.

Dalai Lama (XIV) [Tenzin Gyatso] and Jeffery Hopkins. *The Kalachakra Tantra.* Boston: Wisdom Publications, 1985.

Dhal, Upendra Nath. *Goddess Lakshmi: Origin and Development*. Delhi, India: Eastern Book Linkers, 1995.

Dimmitt, Cornelia, and J. A. Buitenan, eds. *Classical Hindu Mythology*. Philadelphia: Temple University Press, 1978.

Dowson, John. *A Classical Dictionary of Hindu Mythology and Religion*. Calcutta, India: 1982.

Eisler, Riane. *The Chalice and the Blade*. San Francisco: Harper & Row, 1988.

Gimbutas, Marija. *The Language of the Goddess*. Berkeley: University of California Press, 1989.

————. *The Living Goddess*. Berkeley: University of California Press, 1999.

Gottner-Abendroth, Heidi. *The Goddess and Her Heros*. Stow, Mass.: Anthony Publishing Company, 1995.

Gupta, Sanjukta. *Laksmi Tantra*. Leiden, Netherlands: Brill, 1972.

Harding, Elizabeth U. *Kali—the Black Goddess of Dakshineswar*. York Beach, Maine: Nicholas-Hays, Inc., 1993.

Harshananda, Swami. *Hindu Gods and Goddesses*. Mysore, India: Sri Ramakrishna Ashrama, 1982.

Hawley, John Stratton, and Donna Maire Wulff, eds. *The Divine Consort: Radha and the Goddesses of India*, Delhi, India: Motilal Banarsidassm, 1984.

————. *DEVI—Goddesses of India*. Berkeley and Los Angeles: University of California Press, 1996.

Integral Yoga Institute, compiler. *Dictionary of Sanskrit Names*. Yogaville, Va.: Integral Yoga Publications, 1989.

Kinsley, David. *Hindu Goddesses*. Berkeley and Los Angeles: University of California Press, 1988.

Monaghan, Patricia. *The Goddess Path*. St. Paul, Minn.: Llewellyn Publications, 1999.

————. *Goddesses and Heroines*. St. Paul, Minn.: Llewellyn Publications, 1997.

Pargiter, F. Eden, B.A. *The Markandeya Purana*. Delhi, India: Asiatic Society of Bengal, 1981.

Pinchman, Tracy. *The Rise of the Goddess in the Hindu Tradition*. Albany: State University of New York, 1994.

Ranade, R. D. *Mysticism in India: The Poet-Saints of Maharastra*. Albany: State University of New York Press, 1983.

Rao, Prof. S. K. Ramachandra. *Sri Sukta: Text with Translation and Explanation*. Bangalore, India: Kalpatharu Reseach Academy, 1985.

Stone, Merlin. *When God Was a Woman*. New York: Dial Press, 1976.

Tapasyananda, Swami. *Sri Lalita Shasranama*. Madras, India: Sri Ramakrishna Math, date not indicated.

Vimalandanda, Swami. *Sri Lalithambika Shasranama Stotram*. Tirupparaiturai, India: Sri Ramakrishna Tapovanam, 1985.

Recommended

Feuerstein, Georg. *Tantra—The Path of Ecstasy*. Boston and London: Shambhala, 1998.

Frawley, David. *Tantric Yoga and the Wisdom Goddesses*. Salt Lake City: Passage Press, 1994.

Index

abundance, 79–83, 88, 92–103
action, 19
acupuncture, 13, 239
Adbhuta Ramayana, 132
Aditya Hridaya hymn, 154–55
affirmations, 27–28
Agastya, Sage, 143–55
Ajna Chakra, 239
Akhandananda, Swami, 220, 224
Ammachi, 227–28
Anahata Chakra, 33, 94
Anasuya, 239
appearance, 99
Aquarius, 3–5, 229–30, 239, 249
archetypes, 239
art, 19–20, 34
Arya, 42
Astara, 227
astrology, 239
Atisha, Tibetan Sage, 204–6
Atri, 239
auras, 17–18, 239
Autobiography of a Yogi (Yogananda), 7, 227
Avalokiteshwara, 186–90
    forms of, 197
    stories of Tara, 204
Avalon, Arthur. *See* Woodroffe, Sir John
avatars, 239–40

beads, 237–38
Bernadette, Saint, 192–93
Bhagavan Vishnu, 143
Bhagavata Purana, 130, 173
Bhakti Yoga, 23, 240
Bhanda, 156–57
Bharata, 170, 179

Bharati, 42
Bhija Garbha, 42
Big Bang, 25–26
Bindhu, 159
Blavatsky, H. P., 17
Blofeld, John, 190, 192–93, 199–200
Bodhisattva, 187
Bodhisattva of Compassion: The Mystical Tradition of Kuan Yin (Blofeld), 190, 192–93, 199–200
Bodhisattva Vow, 172, 187–88
Brahma, 35–41, 240
    battle against Mahi Asura, 109–11
    creation of the universe, 29–32
    rising from Kali, 133
    story of Agastya and Lalita, 145
    Yuga (Spiritual Age), 249
Brahma mantras, 73–76
The Brahmananda Purana, 142, 145
The Brahmanas, 34, 240
Brahma Rishis, 86
Brahma Vaivarta, 174
Brahma Vidya, 143
Brahmi, 42
Brahmins, 240
bramacharya, 218
Buddha, 41, 202, 240
    abundance, 79
    incarnation of Vishnu, 180
    Lakshmi's role, 90
Buddha Amitabha, 188–89
Buddhism
    Bodhisattva Vow, 172, 187–88
    compassion, 168
    Eightfold Path, 24
    Gayatri Mantra, 48–50
    Great Mani Mantra, 189–90, 198
    Green Tara, 201–2

Buddhism *(cont.)*
  mantra practice, 12–13
  three jewels of, 202
  White Tara, 202
  The Work, 188
  See also Tibetan Buddhism

Cayce, Edgar, 18–19
chakras, 13–16
  Ajna, 239
  Anahata, 33, 94
  Gayatri Mantra, 49–50
  Kalachakra, 241–42
  location of, 13–14, 27
  Muladhara, 141
  number of, 15
  petals of, 15–16
  piercing of knots, 17
  research and experiments, 14–15
  Soma, 94
  Sri, 145, 156–61
  Swadisthana, 33
Chamundi. *See* Durga-Chamundi
Chandi Path (Satyananda Saraswati),
  228–29
Chandra, 86
Chaney, Earlyne and Robert, 227
chanting, 8, 11–13
charity, 168
Chaura Panchashika, 173
Chenresig. *See* Avalokiteshwara
children, 43–44
Chinese religion
  Avalokiteshwara, 197
  Kuan Yin, 2, 190–94
Christian doctrine, 24
Church of Religious Science, 28
Church of Truth, Pasadena, CA,
  163
Churchward, James, 207–8
Cibique Apache chanting, 11
clairaudience, 15, 19
clairvoyance, 15, 19
classifications of *shakti*, 17–26
communication, 19
compassion, 168, 185–96
  Great Mani Mantra, 198
  Green Tara, 201
  mantras, 188–90
  Tara, Mother of the World, 199–202
  White Tara, 202

concentration, 160
consciousness, 5, 52–53, 76–78, 160
  Sri Chakra, 157–58
  Tara, 201
Cosmic Religion, 197, 228
cows, 42
creation of the universe, 28–32
creativity, 19–20, 127

Daksha, 240
Dalai Lama XIV (Tenzin Gyaltso),
  12–13
Dante, 93
Daya Mata, 226–27
Day in the Life of Brahma, 249
decision making, 19
depression, 161
desires, 160–61
devi, 240
The Devi Mahatmyam, 114–19
Dhameshwari, 42
Dhanvantari, 91–92, 101–2, 240
dharma, 90, 202
Dharmakirti, 205
dimensions of reality, 25–26
disease. *See* healing
The Divine Comedy (Dante), 93
divine love, 168–84, 233–34
Divine Mother, 7, 141
  See also Great Feminine Power
Divine Speech, 31–34
Durga-Chamundi, 105–26, 142, 179–80
  birth of, 106–13
  connection to Kali, 131–32
  defeat of Mahi Asura, 113, 120–22
  The Devi Mahatmyam, 114–19
  mantras of protection, 122–26
  Navaratri festival, 162
  qualities of, 113–20
  unity, 120
Durga Gayatri mantra, 126
Durvasas, 240
Dwapara Yuga, 249

education, 28, 43–44
Eightfold Path, 24
electricity, 20, 127
elements, 157–58
elephants, 86
empathy. *See* compassion
energy bodies. *See chakras*

enlightenment, 48, 187–88
etheric bodies, 240

feminine archetypes, 1
feminine attributes, 6, 157–58
Feminine Trinity, 240
feminism, 1–3
Feuerstein, Georg, 130–31
food, 97
forbidden things, 134
forty-day approach to mantra practice, 235–36
free will, 216

Ganesha, 78
Ganges River, 66, 218–23, 240
Garland of Letters (Woodroffe), 33
Gauri, 145
Gayatri, 37–41, 240
Gayatri Devi, 35–41
Gayatri Mantra, 12, 33–35, 47–51, 240–41
Gita Govinda, 173
granthis, 17, 241
Great Feminine power, 16–26, 140–42
  engagement with the world, 77
  increases in *shakti*, 230–32
  Lalita ceremony, 162–67
  Lalita mantras, 155–56
  Maha Shakti Puja, 162–67
  Navaratri festival, 161–62
  secret doctrine of Sri Vidya, 143–46, 155
  Sri Chakra, 145, 156–61
  story of Agastya, 146–55
  See also *shakti*
Great Fifteen-Syllable Mantra, 138–39
Great Mani Mantra, 189–90, 198
Great Mother, 30–31
Green Tara, 201
Guru Mata, 228
Gurumayi, 227
gurus, 241
  See also teachers

Hatha Yoga, 22–23, 241
Hayagriva, Sage, 143–46, 152, 205, 207
healing, 28, 91–92, 101–2, 230
  Gayatri Mantra, 48
  mantras for protection, 122–26

prana, 19
prema, 172
Healing Mantras (Ashley-Farrand), 11
heart, 94–95
heat, 17–18
Hemavati, 53, 241
Hinn, Benny, 218
Holmes, Ernest, 28
Hsuan Tsang, 204

Iccha Shakti, 19, 52, 106, 127, 241
illness and disease. *See* healing
immortality, 93–94
impatience, 127
Indra, 241
  appearance of Lalita, 156–57
  battle against Mahi Asura, 106–14, 121
  birth of Lakshmi, 83–91
  Durvasas' curse, 83
  Maha Lakshmi Astakam, 91
  Saraswati's curse, 39–41
inner shakti, 21–22
intellectual powers, 18–19
  knowledge, 27–28, 34–35
  memory, 18, 20
  Queen of Knowledge mantra, 45–46
  speech, 27, 31, 32–34
  Tara stories, 206–7
  See also Saraswati

Jesus, 225, 233
Jetsun Ma, 227
Jnana, 241
Jnana Shakti, 18–19, 52, 241
Jnana Yoga, 23

Kala, 128, 130, 159, 241
Kalachakra, 241
Kalachakra Mantra, 12, 242
The Kalachakra Tantra (Tenzin Gyaltso, Dalai Lama XIV), 12–13
Kali, 7, 127–39, 142, 242
  appearance of, 129
  depictions of, 132–34
  Great Fifteen-Syllable Mantra, 138–39
  Iccha Shakti, 127
  interactions with Shiva, 132–33
  Kriya Shakti, 127
  Kundalini Shakti, 127
  the left-hand path, 134

Kali (*cont.*)
  mantras of, 134–39
  praise for, 128
  qualities of, 130–31
  reputation of, 128–32
  story of, 131–37
  transformation from Parvati, 133
  transformation from Sita, 132
  vengeance, 129–30
Kali Puja (Satyananda Saraswati),
    228–29
Kali Yuga, 175, 177–78, 180–81, 242,
    249
Kama, 56–57, 72, 76–77, 242
Kamada Tantra, 128–29
Kama Dhenu, 42
karma, 20, 23–24, 242
  abundance, 81
  nectar of immortality, 94
Karma Yoga, 23, 172, 242
Karunamayi, 228
Kaustubha Gem, 86–87, 90, 242
Kavacha, 242
Kirlean photography, 13
knowledge, 27–28, 34–35
  See also intellectual powers
Krishna, 41, 90
  the *gopis*, 169, 171–72
  love relationships, 169–82
  and Radha, 173–81
  as Rama, 170–73
  story of, 174–81
  wives of, 169–70
Krita Yuga, 249
Kriya Shakti, 19–20, 106, 242
  creativity, 52
  Kali, 127
  Lakshmi, 159–60
  Lalita, 159–60
Kriya Yoga, 23, 242
Kuan Yin, 2, 185–96
  mantra, 194–96
  similarities to Tara, 199–200
  story of, 190–94
  visual depictions of, 199
Kulki, 90
Kumar Rajiva, 190
Kundalini, 242–43
Kundalini Maha Yoga, 228
Kundalini Shakti, 4, 7–8, 20, 127, 243
Kundalini Yoga, 243

Lakshmana, 170, 179, 243
Lakshmi, 30–31, 41, 54–55, 79–104,
    243
  abundance, 79–83, 88–89, 92–95,
    102–3
  appearance in the universe,
    81–83
  battle against Mahi Asura, 106–7,
    110–11
  birth of, 83–93
  creation of Dhanvantari, 91–92
  creation of Radha, 174–81
  emanations of, 152
  immortality, 93–94
  incarnation as Sita and Kali, 132
  killing of King Kamsa, 180
  Kriya Shakti, 159–60
  Lakshmi Tantra, 104
  lotus flower, 94–95
  mantras, 20, 97–103
  names of, 96–97
  Navaratri festival, 162
  power of love, 172, 181–82
  qualities of, 94–97, 100
  scriptures, 81
  seed sounds, 76
  story of Agastya and Lalita, 145
  test of Anasuya, 103–4
Lakshmi Tantra, 81, 104
Lalita, 140–67, 243
  Kriya Shakti, 159–60
  Maha Shakti Puja, 162–67
  mantras, 155–56, 159–61
  Sri Chakra, 156–61
  story of Agastya, 143–55
  See also Great Feminine Power
Lalita Madhava, 173
Lalita Sahasranama, 142, 145, 155,
    163–67
lamas, 243
Lang, Doe, 95–96
Langdharma, Tibetan king, 204
Laya Yoga, 23, 243
the left-hand path, 134
life energy, 19, 21–22
life instructions, 24
light, 17–18, 159
locomotion, 19
Lopamudra, 146–49, 154–55
lotus flower, 94–95, 243
Lotus Sutra, 192–93

love, 232–33
  Krishna, 168–84
  mantras, 182–84
  passion, 56–57, 77, 182

magnetism, 20
Mahabharata, 142–43
Maha Great, 243
Maha Kalpa, 244, 249
Maha Lakshmi, 96
Maha Lakshmi Astakam, 91, 159–60
Maha Nirvana Tantra, 72, 74–75, 128
Maha Shakti Puja, 162–67
Maha Vidya, 42
Mahayuga, 249
Mahi Asura, 106–13, 120–22
malas, 237–38
Malati Madhava, 133
mandala, 197
Manipura Chakra, 244
Manjushri, 46, 244
mantras
  for abundance, 96–103
  Brahma mantras, 73–76
  for compassion, 188–90
  for divine love, 234
  Durga Gayatri mantra, 126
  Gayatri Mantra, 240–41
  Great Fifteen-Syllable Mantra, 138–39
  Great Mani Mantra, 189–90, 198
  growth of life energy, 21–22
  for healing, 48
  Kalachakra Mantra, 12, 242
  during Kali Yuga, 178
  Kuan Yin Mantra, 194–96
  Lakshmi mantras, 20, 97–103
  Lalita mantras, 155–56, 159–61
  for love, 182–84
  for memory, 20
  mula, 208
  Para mantras, 33
  practice of, 12–13, 138–39, 235–38
  for protection, 122–26
  Queen of Knowledge mantra, 45–46
  for relief from difficult circumstances, 137–38
  Sanjivani Mantra, 246
  Sanskrit language, 11–13
  Saraswati mantras, 20, 43–46
  Shiva mantras, 75–76
  Sri Vidya, 143, 247

Tara mantras, 208–14
  for universal peace, 209
Mantra Shakti, 20–21, 52, 244
Mantra Siddhi, 236–37, 244
Manvantara, 249
Markandeya Purana, 112
Mary, 2
masculine attributes
  consciousness, 5, 53, 157–58, 160
  nurturing, 2
Masculine Trinity, 244
Matrikas, 131
Matsya Purana, 35
Maya, 128
Mbuti Pygmy chanting, 11
Melanesian chanting, 11
memory, 18, 20
Menaka, 244
meru, 237–38
misuse of power, 215–25
monkeys, 206–7
monoblock theory of creation, 25
the moon, 86
mother goddesses, 200–206
  See also Tara
Mount Kailas, 244
mudra, 125, 199
Muktananda, Paramahansa, 7, 140, 227
mula, 208
Muladhara chakra, 141
murtis, 162–63
music, 19–20, 22, 27, 34, 42, 44
mysticism, 44–45
myths and stories, 26

Nada, 33, 159
nadis, 13, 244
Naga, 151
Nandi, 244
Narada, Sage, 180, 246
Narayana, 28–32, 244
  appearance of Lakshmi, 82–83, 87–88
  role of Parvati, 54–55
  story of Agastya and Lalita, 145
Navaratri festival, 161–62
Nectar of Immortality, 82–83, 88, 91–94, 159–60
negative ego, 130
Nigama Kalpataru, 134
Nirvana Tantra, 133
Niyamas, 221

One Year of Brahma, 249
oral traditions, 142–43
outer shakti, 21–22

Padma, 95
Pancha Maha Bhuta, 158
Para, 33, 244
Paramahansa, 245
Para Shakti, 17–18, 106, 244
parents, 43–44
Parvati, 52–78, 245
  appearance of Lakshmi, 85–86, 90–91
  battle against Mahi Asura, 108–9,
    111–12, 121
  Brahma mantras, 73–76
  consciousness, 76–78
  incarnation as Kali, 133
  Maha Nirvana Tantra, 72, 74–75
  role in the universe, 53–55
  story of, 55–72
  story of Agastya and Lalita, 147–55
pashyanti, 33, 245
Paul, Saint, 168
peace, 100–101, 209
personality, 99
philosophy, 44–45
Piccila Tantra, 133–34
Ponder, Catherine, 28
power, 16–26, 215–25
  of nature, 20
  personal, 3–10
practice of mantras, 12–13, 138–39
  beads and *malas*, 237–38
  forty-day approach, 235–36
  Mantra Siddhi, 236–37
  number of repetitions, 236–37
Prajapati, 82, 103–4
prana, 19, 21–22, 245
prayer, 22
prema, 172–73
professional success, 98
prosperity, 28, 97–98
protection, 105–26
  mantras, 122–26
  story of Durga-Chamundi, 106–22
  story of Kali, 131–37
  story of Tara, 201–2
  Tara mantras, 209–14
puranas, 26, 245

Queen of Knowledge mantra, 45–46

Radha, 90, 168–84, 245
  love relationship with Krishna,
    169–70
  in scriptures, 173–74
  story of, 174–81
Rahasya Nama.
  See Lalita Sahasranama
Raja Yoga, 245
Raktabija, 131
Rama, 90, 179, 245
  in Agastya's story, 151–55
  connections to Tara, 207–8
  story of, 170–73
Ramakrishna, Paramahansa, 7, 127,
    130–31, 140
Rama Mata, 228
Ramayana, 170, 206–7
Ravana, 41, 152–53, 245–46
  kidnapping of Lakshmi, 177–78
  kidnapping of Sita, 171
Red Annals, 204, 206
reincarnation, 24
Rig Veda, 34
Rudra, 145
Rukmini, 90, 169, 179, 246

Sad Dharma Pundarika Sutra, 189–90
sadguru, 246
sahaja samadhi, 246
Sai Baba, 20
Sakya Jetsun Chiney Luding, 227
samadhi, 246
samsaras, 141
Sanatana Vishwa Dharma, 197, 228
Sangha, 202
Sanjivani Mantra, 246
Sanskrit language, 11–16
Sant Keshavadas, Sadguru, 6, 50, 228
Sarada Devi, 140
Saraswati, 27–51, 141–42, 246
  Creation of the Universe, 28–32
  Divine Speech, 31
  foundation mantra, 43–44
  Gayatri Devi, 35–41
  Gayatri Mantra, 34
  intellectual powers, 27–28, 34–35,
    43–45
  Lakshmi, 30–31
  manifestations of, 33
  mantras of, 20, 43–46
  Mother of the Vedas, 34

mysticism, 44–45
names of, 42
Navaratri festival, 162
qualities of, 42
Queen of Knowledge mantra, 45–46
scriptural references, 34–35
story of Agastya and Lalita, 145
Tibetan practices, 46
visual depictions of, 34
Sata-patha Brahmana, 33
Sati, 53, 246
satsang, 153, 227
Satyabhama, 169, 179–80, 246
Satyananda Saraswati, Swami, 228–29
Satya Sai Baba, 7, 218
Satya Yuga, 249
science, 45
scriptures, 15, 25, 41
  Adbhuta Ramayana, 132
  Bhagavata Purana, 130, 173
  Brahmananda Purana, 142, 145
  The Brahmanas, 34
  Brahma Vaivarta, 174
  Brahma Vidya, 143
  Chaura Panchashika, 173
  Gita Govinda, 173
  Kamada Tantra, 128–29
  Lakshmi Tantra, 81, 104
  Lalita Madhava, 173
  Lalita Sahasranama, 142, 145, 155,
    164–67
  Mahabharata, 142–43
  Maha Nirvana Tantra, 72, 128
  Malati Madhava, 133
  Markandeya Purana, 112
  Matsya Purana, 35
  Nigama Kalpataru, 134
  Nirvana Tantra, 133
  Piccila Tantra, 133–34
  Ramayana, 170
  Red Annals, 204, 206
  Rig Veda, 34
  Sad Dharma Pundarika Sutra, 189, 190
  Sata-patha Brahmana, 33
  Shri Suktam, 81
  Swadhina Bhartrika, 173
  Ujjivala Nilamani, 173–74
  Vidag Dhamadhava, 173
  The Secret Doctrine (Blavatsky), 17
  The Secrets of Charisma (Lang), 95–96
seed sounds, 76, 160

self-healing, 28
  See also healing
selflessness, 172
Self-Realization Fellowship, 227
service, 225
shakti, 4, 16–27, 246
  classifications, 17–26
  life changes, 226, 231–32
  power, 16–26, 215–25
  self-knowledge, 232
  spiritual authority, 217
  spiritual energy, 230–32
  See also specific *shaktis*, e.g., Iccha
    Shakti
shaktipat, 7
Shaktipat Diksha, 140
Shatrugna, 170, 179
Shiva, 5, 39–41, 53, 246
  appearance of Lakshmi, 83–85, 90–91
  battle against Mahi Asura, 108–12
  foundation mantra, 75–76
  influenced by Parvati, 57–72, 77
  interactions with Kali, 132–33
  praise for Kali, 128–29
  role in the universe, 54–56
  story of Agastya, 146–55
  teachings to Parvati, 74–75
Shiva Bala Yogi, 220–24
Shree Ma, 228–29
Shri. *See* Lakshmi
Shri Suktam, 81
Siddha Yoga Foundation, 227
siddhis, 215, 220–22, 247
Sita, 41, 90, 132, 170–73, 247
Situ, 151–53
Soma chakra, 94
sound (*Nada*), 33, 159
Sounds True, 228
speech, 27, 31–34
spiritual growth, 15, 28, 34, 141
  authority, 217
  awakening of kundalini, 23
  consciousness, 52–53
  demonstrations of personal power, 7
  gender, 5–6, 226–29
  Lakshmi's role, 93–95
  Saraswati mantras, 44–45
Sri Anandi Ma, 228
Sri Aurobindo, 140
Sri Chakra, 145, 156–61
Sri Vidya, 143, 247

Sri Yantra, 145, 156–61
Subramanya, 66, 77–78, 247
swadha, *swaha*, and *swara*, 111
Swadhina Bhartrika, 173
Swadisthana Chakra, 33, 247

tantra, 1–2, 131–34, 247
Tantra: Path of Ecstasy (Feuerstein),
    130–31
Tara, 90, 197–214
    Homage to Tara prayer, 212–13
    mantras, 208–14
    mudras, 199
    qualities of, 200–206
    similarities to Kuan Yin, 199–200
    stories of, 206–7
    Tibetan role, 204–6
    visual depictions of, 199
teachers, 230
    spiritual authority, 217
    women as, 226–29
Ten Commandments, 24, 221
Tenzin Gyaltso, Dalai Lama XIV,
    12–13
Teresa (Mother), of Calcutta, 229
thanka, 197
third eye, 202
Tibetan Buddhism
    Avalokiteshwara's feminine form, 197
    branches of, 205–6
    Great Mani Mantra, 189–90
    Homage to Tara prayer, 212–13
    Manjushri, 46, 244
    Para mantra, 33
    Red Annals, 204, 206
    role of Tara, 200–206
    Saraswati, 46
    teaching of Tara, 204–6
    thanka, 197
    tummo, 18
time (*Kala*), 128, 130, 159, 241
Treta Yuga, 249
Tr'itsun, 204
truthfulness, 101
tummo, 18, 247

Uddhava, 181, 247
Ujjivala Nilamani, 173–74
Uma, 53, 247
understanding, 18–19

unity, 78, 120
Unity Church, 28
the universe
    dualist nature of, 82–83
    immortality, 82–83, 88, 93–94
    levels of, 47
    Sri Chakra, 156–61
    story of creation, 29–32
    theories of creation, 25–26
Upaguru, 247–48
upamshu, 33, 248
Upanishads, 15, 248
Uttarkashi, India, 218–23

Vach, 32–34, 42, 248
varuna, 248
vedanta, 248
Vedas, 15, 25–26, 248
vengeance, 129–30
vibhuti, 7, 218, 228, 248
Vidag Dhamadhava, 173
vidya, 248
Vijaya Dasami, 162
vishatkare, 111
Vishnu, 38–41, 54–55, 142, 248
    appearance of Lakshmi, 85–91
    battle against Mahi Asura, 106–14
    creation of Radha, 174–82
    emanations of, 143, 152
    incarnation as Buddha, 180
    Parvati's story, 69–70
    rising from Kali, 133
Vishwamitra, 248–49

Water Bearer, 4–5
Wen Cheng Kung Chu, 204
will, 127
wisdom, 18–19, 201
    See also intellectual powers
women's movement, 1–3, 226–29
Woodroffe, Sir John, 33, 72
written works. *See* scriptures

yajna, 111, 249
Yamas, 221
yoga, 22–23, 172, 249
Yogananda, Paramahansa, 7, 23,
    140–41, 226–27
Yoga Spiritual Age, 249
Yoga Sutras of Patanjali, 15, 249

About the Author

THOMAS ASHLEY-FARRAND (Namadeva) practiced mantra-based spiritual disciplines since 1973 and was an acknowledged expert in Sanskrit mantra spiritual disciplines. Vedic Priest, author, and international lecturer and storyteller, Mr. Ashley-Farrand made presentations in the U.S. and Canada as well as India. He was priest-in-residence for the Temple of Cosmic Religion in Washington, D.C., from 1973 to 1980. Thomas lived in Southern California, with his wife, Satyabhama, an attorney in private practice, who often performed the ancient Vedic ceremonies with him. He died in 2010.

www.sanskritmantra.com.